Pregnancy
The Miracle Journey

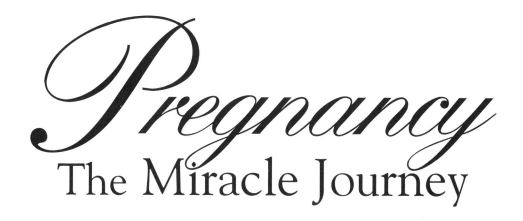

Pregnancy
The Miracle Journey

Jessica Lee Kelly

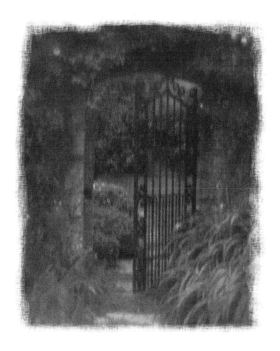

Herald
Press

Scottdale, Pennsylvania
Waterloo, Ontario

Library of Congress Cataloging-in-Publication Data
Kelly, Jessica Lee, 1965-
    Pregnancy : the miracle journey / Jessica Lee Kelly.
        p.   cm.
    ISBN 0-8361-9088-2 (alk. paper)
    1. Pregnant women—Prayer-books and devotions—English.
2. Pregnancy—Religious aspects—Christianity. I. Title.
BV4847.K45 1999
242'.6431—dc21   98-45340

The paper used in this publication is recycled and meets the minimum requirements of the American National Standard for Information Sciences—Permanence of Paper for Printed Library Materials, ANSI Z39.48-1984.

Credits for other quotations are listed on page 6.

PREGNANCY: THE MIRACLE JOURNEY
Copyright © 1999 by Herald Press, Scottdale, Pa. 15683
        Published simultaneously in Canada by Herald Press,
        Waterloo, Ont. N2L 6H7. All rights reserved
        Herald Press Web Site: www.mph.org
Library of Congress Catalog Card Number: 98-45340
International Standard Book Number: 0-8361-9088-2
Book and cover design by Merrill R. Miller
Photographs from Corel Photo Gallery

08 07 06 05 04 03 02 01 00 99 10 9 8 7 6 5 4 3 2 1

To my precious Lord,
for the blessings of miracles.
From my mother,
Sharon,
to my sons,
Colton and Clayton,
"May the circle be unbroken."

Credits

Special thanks to these women, who graciously gave me permission to quote them:

Name	Week
Christine Ritmo	7
Sheila Morales	9
Debbie Boyd	10, 19
Sandy Wright	11
Julie Frisbie	12
Kate Farrell	13
Melodee M. Young	14
Rebecca D. Hayslip	15
Martha Robuck	17
Barbara (Barbie) Johnson Reilly	18
Laurie McClure	22
Deborah Dee Grizzard	23
Bren Turk	26
Linda Davis	28
Linda Werner	29
Anita Gustafson	30
Tracy Roberts	32
Jo Ann Dickinson	37
Lisa B. Stickney	38
Freyja Carlstedt	39
Sharon Lee	40

Kate Farrell's quoted piece (week 13) is from *Art and Love: An Illustrated Anthology of Love Poetry*, from The Metropolitan Museum of Art, New York, and published by Bulfinch Press, a division of Little, Brown, & Company, Boston, 1992.

Melodee M. Young credits some of her thoughts (week 14) to things learned in Bible Study Fellowship International.

Contents

The hand of God reaches out,
and two become one.
The spark of life,
so tiny,
so precious,
so wondrous,
divides and redoubles,
builds and forms.
Selecting from generations, God recreates,
taking you on a Miracle Journey.

The Pilgrim: _____

The Journey started on _____

The Journey was completed on _____

The Miracle is named _____

O Lord, I beg you, . . .
teach us how to bring up the child who is to be born.
–Judges 13:8, NIV

Foreword

*T*HE process of conception, fetal development, and birth is indeed a miracle to behold. Even after a decade of having had the honor of participating in the births of several thousand babies, I remain awed and moved by the beauty and magnificence of the entire process.

Jessica Lee Kelly guides the reader along *The Miracle Journey*, beginning with the embryonic period, the third week after ovulation and fertilization, which begins the first month. This is the fifth week from the start of the last menstrual period. She captures the emotional and spiritual developments of pregnancy. Her book uses a format that allows the reader to gain insight into these changes and to analyze them more completely.

The author addresses physiological and psychological changes during the nine-month pregnancy in a beautifully summarized fashion. Nutritional and exercise recommendations are made for general consideration. For specific medical questions or concerns, the reader can refer to the numerous medical information books available. As with any type of medical advice, the mother should discuss her particular situation with her physician.

Jessica Lee Kelly has done a remarkable job of helping the reader with motherhood preparation by exploring topics dealing with emotional and spiritual growth during pregnancy. This is a unique book and one that is overdue. I will definitely use this book in my practice, as a gift to my patients for their enjoyment and benefit.

—*Angelo C. Mendez, M.D.*
Fellow of the American College of Obstetrics and Gynecology

Preface

*T*HE *Miracle Journey* was designed as a journal within a book of relevant and timely essays and Bible verses. Pregnancy, like life, is a journey made of memorable moments:

The plus on the pregnancy test.

The first morning you woke up and *didn't* get sick.

The Saturday you lost your waist and thus your ability to wear jeans.

The car ride when you felt the first kick.

The night you flushed eight times.

The burp that broke your water.

The birthing cry when your miracle was born.

These moments don't have to be noted on paper for a mother to remember. But spiritual stretching, growth of faith, and Christ-clinging closeness occur over time. They are not always things we can readily put our finger on for timely exactness. These moments are blended into the gray areas of life, when we are just putting one foot in front of the other and walking toward tomorrow.

I've found that writing in a journal is an excellent way for Christians to experience God. Noting your prayers, praises, daily trials, and testimonies allows you opportunities to see the living God working specifically in your life. You can look back on the day, week, month, and year, and start to see the picture God is forming. An event finally makes sense, another connects, images form, prayers of yesterday match answers of today, and faith is built.

Faith, that invisible foundation of your life, can be confirmed by your own written words: Today God was there, and there, and here. God did this, and this, and even that. In your journal is the record: I asked, God answered. I needed, God provided. I made a mess, God handed me the mop. Wow! God cares. God loves me. God disciplines me. God blesses me. God keeps his promises.

Pregnancy is one of the most exciting times of a woman's life. It is also a time of great change and anxious expectancy. The road to motherhood is not easy. Yet it is a valuable time of preparation that should be seized with both spiritual hands, for parenting is one of the greatest tasks God gives us. Therefore, we must come prepared and be fortified with faith.

Keeping a journal builds faith. Such writing does not have to be time-consuming and detailed. It can be simple lists: "I ate, I did, I felt, I weighed, I need, baby was . . ." It can be brief notes like these: "Thanks, Lord, for the front-row parking space today at the grocery store. My swollen ankles needed it." Or, "I heard God's voice today. As the sun set in a brilliant, fiery watercolor, God whispered, 'I love you.' "

As you log your journey in this journal, you are making word pictures that describe what is happening to you day by day and what God is doing in your life. If this book does not give you enough room, you can expand your writing in a companion notebook.

Once finished, *The Miracle Journey* is a panorama proclaiming the work of God's hands in the spiritual growth of a woman. Faith is built during this journey called motherhood.

I know the one in whom I have put my trust,
and I am sure that he is able to guard until that day what I have entrusted to him.
Hold to the standard of sound teaching that you have heard from me,
in the faith and love that are in Christ Jesus.
Guard the good treasure entrusted to you,
with the help of the Holy Spirit living in us.
—2 Timothy 1:12-14

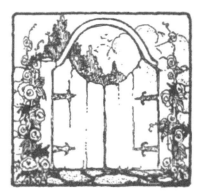

CONGRATULATIONS! You're pregnant! God's life-giving hand has touched you, blessing you with the miraculous privilege of producing a new life.

Already you've taken the first steps along a path countless women have walked before you. You've set off on the Miracle Journey. Yet your journey is unique—it is yours.

Your journey is indeed a miracle. It is awe-inspiring, metamorphosing, and exciting.

Begin by thinking of yourself as a pilgrim, embarking on a holy mission. You are traveling toward a destination, changing mind, body, and soul as you go forward with every step.

You Are Prepared

Within your body is a built-in road map, drafted by the Creator God. You study the bodily process of pregnancy, preparing yourself for the road ahead. You know there will be hills and valleys, tears and laughter, days of drudgery and days of great joy.

You Plan

With a map and compass, you plot your travel plans along a course that will take about 280 days to complete. Navigating ensures smooth sailing, even through the roughest waters.

You Set Goals

Goals give the traveler a sense of direction when faced with turbulent emotions, vague anxieties, and mounting discomforts. Goals keep you focused on the vision, and achievement brings encouragement and growth.

You Record Your Journey

By pointing out landmarks along the way, you can see how far you've come. Keeping a journal helps you recognize God's presence. When you look back, you clearly see God's guidance, love, discipline, and blessings in your daily walk with him (also see page 16).

How to Use This Planner

Doctors date pregnancy from the first day of your last menstrual period, so we begin this journal at week 5. This is just weeks after ovulation and fertilization. You will chronicle each step of your journey, detailing your feelings, diet, exercise, prayers, praises, and appointments on a daily basis. No ache, pain, pound, inch, change, occurrence, annoyance, emotion, or event is too small. Record them daily, and recap the theme of the week in "My Record of Faith," on page 111. When your journey is complete, you have a detailed guide for the next pregnancy and a priceless keepsake for yourself and your child. Once finished, *The Miracle Journey* is a tool for seeing God's work in a life. It is a record of prayers and answers, fears and courage, and the growth of a woman's faith as she journeys toward motherhood.

A journey of a thousand leagues begins with the first step.
—Lao-tzu

Thus says the Lord: Stand at the crossroads, and look, and ask for the ancient paths, where the good way lies; and walk in it, and find rest for your souls.
—Jeremiah 6:16

The First Trimester

Being Prepared

Take care of important business right away.

Decide on a prenatal care-provider, and make your first appointment.

Confirm your health insurance and learn about your coverage (see page 120).

Confirm your company's maternity-leave policy. Decide how much time you will take off.

Become aware of your environment.

Stay away from people with contagious diseases.

Tell anyone working on your body (dentist, chiropractor, fitness trainer), "I'm pregnant!"

Stop habits that harm the fetus: smoking and using alcohol, drugs, caffeine, sugar substitutes.

Don't just settle for anything. Find out what's *best* for *you.*

Research. Read up on what's ahead. Buy, borrow, or check out a good pregnancy reference book. Ask your doctor to recommend one.

Planning and Doing

A Healthy You

Do the diet drill and find out where your diet is deficient (see pages 116-117).

With your doctor's help, decide on an exercise program. Plan those crucial workouts into your weekly schedule (see pages 118-119).

A Smart Steward

Decide how much maternity leave you will take. Begin planning the finances and schedule for it.

Figure out what your medical expenses will be and begin budgeting for them (see pages 120-124).

Prepare a baby budget and begin a savings program (see pages 122-124).

Start dreaming and saving for your second-trimester last-fling vacation.

Childcare

If you plan to work away from home, begin thinking about childcare options. If there is a childcare facility you know you want to use, put your name on the waiting list now. If not, start networking to find one.

Goal-Setting

Reconfirm the lifestyle changes you will promise on week 5.

Set a weekly exercise goal.

Set a weekly savings goal to pay for birth-related expenses.

Keeping a Journal

Record each day of your journey by describing the changes taking place in your body, emotions you are feeling, situations that occurred, foods you ate, how you exercised, if you had sex, medications you took, and how you slept. Write down the names of the people you told the good news to. Record all the good and not-so-good advice you're beginning to accumulate.

Along the way, take pictures of the changes in your body.

Pages 126-128 are provided for "More Journal Notes" as you reflect on your pregnancy, your faith, and your friends and family accompanying you on this Miracle Journey.

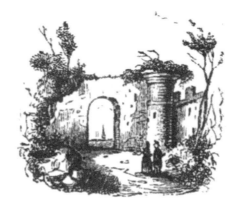

First Month

Weeks 5~8

Prayer for the Child

O Lord, our child is but an embryo, with tiny head and trunk. During this month, you will form the beginning of its features. Bless each of the tiny limb buds, which will grow into arms and legs. Create hands that will later serve you, and strong legs that will lead our precious child to your narrow path. You have formed our little one's heart, and on day 25, it began beating for the first time. Bless this tiny soul, that this dear one may grow to be a child after your own heart. Amen.

Prayer for the Mother

O Lord, I'm pregnant. Wow! I look at myself in wonderment and a sense of disbelief. On the outside, my body looks the same as before. But inside, I know things are moving, shaking, growing, and changing. My hormones, progesterone and estrogen, are sending me on a roller-coaster ride, emotionally and physically.

I feel _____ (tired, nauseated, emotional, overwhelmed, excited, joyous, scared).

Help me to take one day at a time. Help me to choose joy each day and to realize I have been truly blessed. This is the day that you have made, Lord. Let me rejoice and be glad in it. Amen.

Theme of the Month: Miracles

Do you realize that miracles happen every day? Birth is an ordinary, everyday event, but when you become part of the process, it takes on new meaning. Start looking for the subtle gifts God gives you each day. Be watchful and thankful. Every day, record five special things God did for you. It will help you choose joy and will give you zest to grow the fruit of the Spirit.

Bible Study

This month, study the story of Hannah, found in 1 Samuel 1:1—2:21. Write your own personal prayer of praise for the blessing the Lord has given you in this still-tiny miracle of a child.

For this child I prayed.
—1 Samuel 1:27

A hand rests protectively on a flat belly,
and a voice whispers to the world, "I am."
A slow smile blossoms with our joy.
We look to the horizon, embarking on a journey,
anticipating that our lives will change,
wondering, preparing, planning—
already in love.

WHETHER this was an anticipated event or one that came as a complete surprise, today you must make new commitments to yourself and chart the best course for the completion of your Miracle Journey. The first step is to change your lifestyle. Make new resolutions of change to improve your chances for a healthy baby.

Finding your motivation to change is easy—you're pregnant!

Change today by promising out loud:

I resolve to stop habits that would harm the fetus—smoking and using alcohol or recreational drugs.

I resolve to eat nutritious meals and increase fluid intake.

I resolve to exercise and practice relaxation exercises.

I resolve to get more rest and reduce stress.

I resolve to keep my doctor's appointments and educate myself on the pregnancy process.

I resolve to be prepared and plan for the future.

I resolve to set goals and record the results.

I resolve to set boundaries and say no when my health and baby must come first.

I resolve to pray daily for our child and the new family being created.

Do what is right
as a sacrifice to the Lord
and trust the Lord.
—Psalm 4:5, NCV

Day 1

Put these things into practice, devote yourself to them, so that all may see your progress. *1 Timothy 4:15*

Day 2

The Lord possessed me in the beginning of his way, before his works of old. *Proverbs 8:22, KJV*

Day 3

In the beginning was the Word, and the Word was with God, and the Word was God. . . . All things came into being through him, and without him not one thing came into being. *John 1:1, 3*

Day 4

Now the man knew his wife Eve, and she conceived and bore Cain, saying, "I have produced a man with the help of the Lord." *Genesis 4:1*

Day 5

I praise you, for I am fearfully and wonderfully made. Wonderful are your works; that I know very well. *Psalm 139:14*

Day 6

And you will say in that day: Give thanks to the Lord, call on his name; make known his deeds among the nations; proclaim that his name is exalted. *Isaiah 12:4*

Day 7

Sing praises to the Lord, for he has done gloriously; let this be known in all the earth. *Isaiah 12:5*

I applied my mascara by toilet-bowl reflection,
commuted to work with airsickness bags between my legs,
and ticked off the minutes of my first trimester with saltine crackers.
I had never felt so gloriously miserable in my life.

"IT'S not easy bein' green," sings Kermit the Frog, and most of us readily agree. For a majority of women, pregnancy arrives with flu-like symptoms. You feel run-down, off kilter, and always nauseated. As you wonder when your "late period" will arrive , alas, you start to wonder, *Do I have the flu, . . . or a fetus!*

By now you've concluded that these telltale signs are your body's way of dealing with the tremendous upheavals—pardon the pun—that are occurring inside your newly pregnant body. Contrary to its name, morning sickness can occur at any time of day (or all day) and may last days, weeks, or months. In addition, so-called morning sickness is not a disease. The discomforts of pregnancy generally come from the body adjusting to its task of creating a new life rather than from a failure of the body.

Although the cause of morning sickness is not known, most experts believe the high level of the pregnancy hormone HCG found in the bloodstream during the first trimester is likely responsible for your distress. If you are experiencing significant morning sickness and vomiting that causes weight loss and possible dehydration, call your physician immediately. For such cases, there are medications for nausea and vomiting.

If you're suffering, eat often, even before you feel hungry, nibbling a little all day. Avoid anything that might make one of your five senses queasy. Keep snacks stashed in your handbag, car, desk drawer, and on your nightstand. Being prepared can be a remedy in itself.

The only cure for morning sickness seems to be time. For some of you, it will stop when you reach week 12; others will continue to suffer to the end. If you find yourself looking at your reflection in the toilet several times a day, smile and tell your reflection that this is a reassuring sign that your body is hard at work producing a new life.

Do not fear, for I am with you,
do not be afraid, for I am your God;
I will strengthen you, I will help you,
I will uphold you with my victorious right hand.
—Isaiah 41:10

Day 1

Sustain me with raisins, refresh me with apples; for I am faint with love. *Song of Solomon 2:5*

_____
_____
_____

Day 2

Be strong, and let your heart take courage, all you who wait for the Lord. *Psalm 31:24*

_____
_____
_____

Day 3

My soul melts for heaviness: strengthen me according to your word. *Psalm 119:28, KJV, adapted*

_____
_____
_____

Day 4

It is better to suffer for doing good, if suffering should be God's will, than to suffer for doing evil. *1 Peter 3:17*

_____
_____
_____

Day 5

Answer me when I pray to you, my God who does what is right. Make things easier for me when I am in trouble. Have mercy on me and hear my prayer. *Psalm 4:1, NCV*

_____
_____
_____

Day 6

After you have suffered for a little while, the God of all grace, who has called you to his eternal glory in Christ, will himself restore, support, strengthen, and establish you. *1 Peter 5:10*

_____
_____
_____

Day 7

I applied my heart to what I observed and learned a lesson from what I saw. *Proverbs 24:32, NIV*

_____
_____
_____
_____

21

*T*was the world's worst when it came to eating a balanced diet. I hated vegetables. My spoiled taste buds didn't want anything "good for you." When I began to think about conception and pregnancy, I had to alter my choices in the cafeteria line dramatically. It wasn't easy to choose corn over corn chips or a fruit cup instead of my favorite cookies. I struggled daily and endured with distaste each of the four to five servings of vegetables I forced myself to consume. But I knew there was a tiny being totally dependent on me for its nourishment. Giving our baby the best opportunity to be born healthy was directly tied to what I ate—along with my weight gain and chances for stretch marks. I needed help to change my bad lifestyle habit of unbalanced and unhealthy eating, so I talked with a dietitian, who taught me three simple principles.

Make every bite count. Some things provide only empty calories for baby: a soda has caffeine, sodium, and sugar or Nutrasweet. Milk, fruit juice, or just plain water is a much more nutritious choice. All calories are not created equal, so choose with care what will most benefit baby.

Eating for two doesn't allow you twice the calories. How many calories should you eat? Make a good estimate by taking your weight before pregnancy and multiplying it by 15. Thus, for example, 130 pounds times 15 = 1950 calories per day. During pregnancy you need only about 300 more calories a day than in your normal diet. You can get 300 calories in just two glasses of milk.

To assure yourself a well-balanced diet, focus on the four basic food groups:

Fruits and vegetables

Fight infection, promote healthy skin, and provide vitamins and minerals. You need four or more servings each day. Choose at least one serving rich in vitamin A, such as vegetables with green leaves. Select at least one serving rich in vitamin C, such as citrus fruit.

Whole-grain bread and cereal

Provide energy, add fiber to avoid constipation, and help reduce morning sickness. Include a variety of complex carbohydrates. You need four or more servings daily.

Dairy products

Aid growth of new tissue and repair body cells. You need four or more servings daily. If you don't get enough calcium, baby will steal it from your bones, setting you up for osteoporosis (soft bones) later in life. So drink your milk, and if you don't like milk, substitute other dairy items such as yogurt or cheese.

Meat, poultry, fish, nuts, beans

Provide protein, iron, and vitamins. You need three or more servings each day. If you suffer from anemia, make sure to eat red meat for at least one serving.

You are what you eat, and so will be baby.
—Christine Ritmo

22

O taste and see that the Lord is good; happy are those who take refuge in him.
—Psalm 34:8

Day 1

Go, eat your food with gladness, and drink your drink with a joyful heart, for it is now that God favors what you do. *Ecclesiastes 9:7, NIV*

_____

_____

Day 2

As an apple tree among the trees of the wood, so is my beloved among young men. With great delight I sat in his shadow, and his fruit was sweet to my taste. *Song of Solomon 2:3*

_____

_____

Day 3

Through him, then, let us continually offer a sacrifice of praise to God, that is, the fruit of our lips that confess his name. *Hebrews 13:15*

_____

_____

Day 4

Do not work for the food that perishes, but for the food that endures for eternal life, which the Son of Man will give you. For it is on him that God the Father has set his seal. *John 6:27*

_____

_____

Day 5

Wherefore I pray you to take some meat: for this is for your health. *Acts 27:34, KJV*

_____

_____

Day 6

For the kingdom of God is not food and drink but righteousness and peace and joy in the Holy Spirit. *Romans 14:17*

_____

_____

Day 7

You need milk! *Hebrews 5:12*

_____

_____

God has made everything beautiful in its time.
He has also set eternity in the hearts of all;
yet they cannot fathom what God has done from beginning to end.
—Ecclesiastes 3:11, NIV, adapted

Paste here a favorite
full-length photo
of yourself
before pregnancy,
or take a new picture
today
and use that.

You Are Beautiful!

Today, _____,
I can look behind me and see the first footsteps of the Miracle Journey.
I can look at myself here and see my body the way it's been,
and the way it will be again when the journey is complete.
I can look ahead, anticipating the awesome changes that my body will go through
as it creates our child.
I am beautiful!

Day 1

God saw everything that he had made, and indeed, it was very good. And there was evening and there was morning, the sixth day. *Genesis 1:31*

_____

_____

Day 2

You are beautiful, . . . my love. *Song of Solomon 6:4*

_____

_____

Day 3

Let your father and mother be glad; let her who bore you rejoice. *Proverbs 23:25*

_____

_____

Day 4

Who is this that appears like the dawn, fair as the moon, bright as the sun, majestic as the stars in procession? *Song of Solomon 6:10, NIV*

_____

_____

Day 5

I will satisfy the weary, and all who are faint I will replenish. *Jeremiah 31:25*

_____

_____

Day 6

"The two will become one flesh." So they are no longer two, but one. *Mark 10:8, NIV*

_____

_____

Day 7

Every moving thing that lives shall be food for you; and just as I gave you the green plants, I give you everything. *Genesis 9:3*

_____

_____

Pop quiz: What did you eat today? Did you balance your diet from the four basic food groups? Eat an extra helping of vegetables, and then treat yourself to your favorite yogurt or ice cream.

_____

_____

_____

Second Month

Weeks 9~12

Prayer for the Child

Our child is now a fetus with all the major body organs and systems forming and developing. Your hand, O great Creator, is molding ears, ankles, and tiny wrists, as fingers and toes finish blooming. Your loving hand forms small eyelids, which you seal shut until later. The first bone cells are manufactured within your growing miracle. My placenta, the channel through which oxygen, nutrients, drugs, hormones, and other substances pass from me to baby, is present and working. What a wondrous body you have given me in which to produce a child. I am so thankful to be called "Woman, taken out of man, bone of my husband's bone, and flesh of his flesh" (Genesis 2:23, adapted). I praise you for motherhood, your unique gift to women. In this child, two truly have become one. Your precious gift to us is now a little over one inch long but weighs less than an ounce. Bless this tiny, helpless, vulnerable life with growth and health within me. Amen.

Prayer for the Mother

I'm so tired, Lord. I know the total volume of blood in my body has increased to feed the growing baby, and inside I am a high-powered baby-making factory. But I don't really *feel* pregnant yet, just run-down and tired. Help me persevere through this first trimester, when I must give so much of myself to something I can't even feel inside of me. Help me to eat what is right and to take care of your precious baby and myself. Make me into the mother that you would have me be today. Let me stand firm in the resolutions I made to change my lifestyle so I can offer my best to this baby. Amen.

Planning. The Theme for the Month Is *Plan, Plan, Plan!*

Because you're too tired to do much of anything else, start thinking about the important decisions you will be making down the road. Consider coming expenses, complete your baby budget, and start saving today (see pages 120-124). Start thinking about other decisions dealing with maternity leave, childcare, prenatal testing, and moving or remodeling your home to make room for baby. Stop by a travel agency and dream a little about a destination for a last-fling vacation.

Bible Study

This month, study the story of Sarah found in Genesis, chapters 16, 18, and 21. Notice what a great thing God does with Sarah's laughing disbelief. What a wonderful sense of humor the almighty God has! What gifts has God given you along with your pregnancy?

_____
_____
_____
_____
_____
_____
_____
_____
_____
_____
_____
_____
_____
_____
_____
_____
_____
_____
_____
_____
_____

Sarah conceived and bore Abraham a son in his old age, at the time of which God had spoken to him. Abraham gave the name Isaac ["he laughs"] to his son whom Sarah bore him. Now Sarah said, "God has brought laughter for me; everyone who hears will laugh with me."
—Genesis 21: 2-3, 6

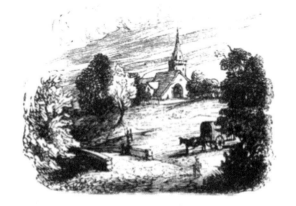

I wanted to tell the world our wonderful news. The waiting was hard; we were so excited.
But treasuring it privately gave us an intimacy we'd never shared before.
Announcing our joy at the start of the second trimester was worth the wait.
We glowed with the words.
—Sheila Morales

So . . . you're pregnant!

What was your initial response when the test came back positive? Joy, disbelief, excitement, trepidation, anxiety? Some of you probably felt like running through the streets to proclaim the joyous news to anyone! You probably kissed your husband and called your best friend and your parents. Maybe you sank to your knees, realizing the enormous life-changing event that had already taken place and the change and responsibility you had to accept. I'm certain several of you went completely numb with denial, disbelief, and shock. Some of you probably said a silent prayer, asking that this pregnancy would "stick," holding back joy until you knew for sure.

Pregnant women have varied reactions to the news, and so will others. Your mate, parents, friends, and co-workers will each look at your big announcement from different angles. Your husband might be so excited that he can't wait to remodel a room for the baby. Other fathers-to-be might view children as a responsibility that will force them finally to grow up and work with their partners in providing a secure home. Your parents might feel too young to be called grandparents, or they might be delighted to welcome a new child into the family.

Single or childless friends might think that once the baby comes, you will be too busy for them. Some might be resentful, others jealous. On the other hand, those friends might hope they can be "aunts" and "uncles" to your children. Bosses and co-workers will probably be pleased to hear your news. However, a few might view a pregnancy as nine months of frequent absenteeism and poor performance. Some might assume that you'll resign after your maternity leave. Others will support you in making the best decision for your family.

You and your mate will think the whole world should celebrate your pregnancy, but the whole world has its own agenda. Be prepared for a variety of reactions to your news. Before you tell people, think about how they will react. Preparing yourself helps safeguard your own feelings and your hormonally turbulent emotions. Only *you* and your husband can decide who and when to tell. The great thing about the Miracle Journey is that you can keep the big news a secret for several months.

It is most important that you and your husband honor God's blessing by deciding that being pregnant is GOOD NEWS. A miracle is taking place. This joy is worth shouting from the mountaintops. God's very hand has touched your lives and blessed you. Your miracle is good news.

How beautiful upon the mountains are the feet of the messenger who announces peace, who brings good news, who announces salvation, who says to Zion,
"Your God reigns."
—Isaiah 52:7

Day 1

Then I will thank you in the great congregation; in the mighty throng I will praise you. *Psalm 35:18*

_____

_____

_____

Day 2

Likewise all to whom God gives wealth and possessions and whom he enables to enjoy them, and to accept their lot and find enjoyment in their toil—this is the gift of God. *Ecclesiastes 5:19*

_____

_____

_____

Day 3

For we are what he has made us, created in Christ Jesus for good works, which God prepared beforehand to be our way of life. *Ephesians 2:10*

_____

_____

_____

Day 4

Then I will go to the altar of God, to God my exceeding joy; and I will praise you with the harp, O God, my God. *Psalm 43:4*

_____

_____

_____

Day 5

Every generous act of giving, with every perfect gift, is from above, coming down from the Father of lights, with whom there is no variation or shadow due to change. *James 1:17*

_____

_____

_____

Day 6

The Lord of hosts says, See if I will not open the windows of heaven for you and pour down for you an overflowing blessing. *Malachi 3:10, adapted*

_____

_____

Day 7

They . . . worshiped God, singing, "Amen! Blessing and glory and wisdom and thanksgiving and honor and power and might be to our God forever and ever! Amen." *Revelation 7:11-12*

_____

_____

WANTED: Individual who will work twenty-four hours a day, seven days a week.
No vacation, no sick leave, no lunch hour, no breaks.
Must have the patience of a saint, nerves of steel, a heart of gold, the attitude of angels.
Salary nonnegotiable. The frail need not apply.
—Debbie Boyd

*D*URING pregnancy, part of you becomes a baby-making machine. As fetal brain cells multiply and primordial buds gradually change into tiny arms and legs, your body is busy manufacturing the baby's life-support system, the placenta, which won't be complete until the third month. As all this creating is going on in the uterus, your control panel—the brain—is trying to adjust and manage all the new physical and emotional demands of the Miracle Journey.

No wonder you're tired! It's no surprise that sometimes you wish you could tell your responsibilities to take a hike so you could crawl into bed until you begin the second trimester. Don't let anybody kid you—the fatigue is *real*. It's time to pull back and say, "No, I can't do that right now." You need to delegate, and let some things go.

You and the baby are the main events. Your health and your unborn child must come first. Repeat this to yourself whenever you're feeling guilty about missing work for a doctor's appointment. You are not a failure because you have failed to cook a single meal all week. It's completely normal to fall asleep thirty minutes into the hot new video you've been dying to see. After all, you are tired, and your pregnant body is demanding extra rest these days.

Inside, you are working twenty-four hours a day to make this baby. During this time, things on the side are extra. Taking care of yourself and the baby is your all-consuming, most-critical, top-priority job. Anything else you do—cleaning, working, mothering, being a wife—must be adapted to fit around that job. As a mother, you must learn to set priorities and conserve your energy, which is being drained by the baby. In the years to come, you will need these skills.

Whatever you do, do your work heartily, as for the Lord rather than for people;
knowing that from the Lord you will receive the reward of the inheritance.
—Colossians 3:23-24, NIV, adapted

Day 1

He said, "My presence will go with you, and I will give you rest." *Exodus 33:14*

_____

_____

Day 2

Six days you shall work, but on the seventh day you shall rest; even in plowing time and in harvest time you shall rest. *Exodus 34:21*

_____

_____

Day 3

For God alone my soul waits in silence; from him comes my salvation. He alone is my rock and my salvation, my fortress; I shall never be shaken. *Psalm 62:1-2*

_____

_____

Day 4

Ascribe to the Lord the glory due his name; bring an offering, and come before him. Worship the Lord in holy splendor; tremble before him, all the earth. The world is firmly established; it shall never be moved. *1 Chronicles 16:29-30*

_____

_____

Day 5

My grace is sufficient for you, for power is made perfect in weakness. *2 Corinthians 12:9*

_____

_____

Day 6

Surely God is my salvation; I will trust, and will not be afraid, for the Lord God is my strength and my might; he has become my salvation. *Isaiah 12:2*

_____

_____

Day 7

Those who wait for the Lord shall renew their strength, they shall mount up with wings like eagles, they shall run and not be weary, they shall walk and not faint. *Isaiah 40:31*

_____

_____

Pop quiz: Are you practicing relaxing? Are you saying no and setting necessary boundaries when needed? Today, restate you resolutions from week 5.

_____

_____

_____

Only six hours before I was to have a hysterectomy, it was discovered that I was "miraculously" pregnant. Midway through the pregnancy, a sonogram showed that the baby had problems and would not live past delivery.
Two months later he was born and lived for one hour in our arms.
We named him Tobie, as it means "the Lord is good." Though grieved, we believed God had been good to allow us the incredible experiences of pregnancy and birth. God has blessed us through adoption with three wonderful children: Jesse, "Gift from God"; Micah Joy, "Like the Lord"; and Zachary, "Jehovah has remembered." Our Lord is good.
—Sandy Wright

GOD'S greatest gift is that he is the same yesterday, today, and tomorrow. He is always good. Even through the worst of situations, when the unthinkable is happening, our God is always good. We can cling to his unshakable character.

Let us remember that sin brought "the sting of death" into our world (1 Corinthians 15:56). Let us hate the enemy—the thief that cheats, lies, and steals away our hopes and dreams. This fallen world offers no guarantees. Our bodies are imperfect. Sometimes a Miracle Journey ends with empty arms. But in loving arms, God holds all our precious ones close in a perfect paradise.

As parents, we do all we can and always have to depend on the Lord to shepherd and care for our children, young or grown. Therefore, we must trust God. With Isaiah, we know that the Lord will feed his flock like a shepherd, gather the lambs into his arms, and carry them in his bosom. He will gently lead the mother sheep (Isaiah 40:11).

The Lord is our Good Shepherd, and he will feed, guide, and shield us. He makes us lie down in new-grown and tender pastures. He leads us to restful, refreshing waters. He gives new life to us, ever leading us in paths of grace and uprightness, for his glorious pleasure.

Yes, dear Lord, we will walk through deep and sunless valleys, but because you are with us, we will not fear or dread evil. Your rod is ever ready to protect, your staff to guide, your faithfulness to comfort. Even in the midst of the unthinkable, you are present to give us what we need today to survive.

You will pour out your Holy Spirit over us to invigorate and refresh us until our souls overflow. Your goodness, mercy, and unfailing love shall follow us all our days, and your presence shall be our dwelling place (Psalm 23).

So let our tears be a love offering to the Giver of life. Like the psalmist, let us cry to the Lord and find comfort by talking things out with trusted friends and counselors (2 Corinthians 1:4). If we have lost a darling baby, we can find new purpose in the family of God, where many would-be parents have a chance to nurture many children (Mark 3:35). Our time on earth is so short. Let our grieving hearts be healed with faith. Let our minds not lean on our own understanding. In the days that come, when we ache with broken hearts and empty arms, let us wait on the Lord and seek him. We know that "the Lord is good," and he will shepherd us forever with his perfect love.

No matter what tomorrow brings, I know my Lord is good.

32

These are the children God has given me. God has been good to me.
—Genesis 33:5, NCV

Day 1

The Lord will feed his flock like a shepherd; he will gather the lambs in his arms, and carry them in his bosom, and gently lead the mother sheep. *Isaiah 40:11, adapted*

_____

_____

_____

Day 2

Though the fig tree does not blossom, and no fruit is on the vines; though the produce of the olive fails and the fields yield no food; though the flock is cut off from the fold and there is no herd in the stalls, yet I will rejoice in the Lord; I will exult in the God of my salvation. *Habakkuk 3:17-18*

_____

_____

_____

Day 3

Trust in the Lord with all your heart, and do not lean on your own understanding. *Proverbs 3:5, NIV*

_____

_____

_____

Day 4

Blessed is anyone who perseveres under trial. Such a one has stood the test and will receive the crown of life that God has promised to those who love him. *James 1:12, NIV and NRSV, adapted*

_____

_____

_____

Day 5

You were wearied by all your ways, but you would not say, "It is hopeless." You found renewal of your strength, and so you did not faint. *Isaiah 57:10, NIV*

_____

_____

Day 6

Those of steadfast mind, you will keep in peace—in peace because they trust in you. *Isaiah 26:3*

_____

_____

Day 7

I, the Lord, am its keeper; every moment I water it. I guard it night and day so that no one can harm it. *Isaiah 27:3*

_____

_____

33

Pregnancy is not accomplished by committee.
Reality is, . . . you walk alone.
—Julie Frisbie

*Y*OUR Miracle Journey might be far different from what you expected it to be. Your mate probably doesn't have sympathy pains. Maybe your family doesn't dote on you. Your closest friend becomes distant. You don't look cute and glow with beauty. Instead, you feel clumsy and fatigued. Your easygoing job takes a nasty turn down Stress Street. Your commute to work is twenty minutes longer because of highway renovations.

You suddenly realize that being pregnant does not get you handicapped parking privileges. Reality sets in quickly. You discover that your idealism has deceived you. You feel hurt, angry, and depressed because you realize that the world does not revolve around your pregnancy.

If the fairy-tale bubble has burst and you are disenchanted, it's time for a quick reality check. Step out of yourself for a moment and try to understand what expectations you have that are not being met. Admit to yourself, "I thought pregnancy was going to be like _____, and it's not." Release your preconceived notions, share your feelings with your mate, and then accept what is real.

No matter how much support the world is giving to your pregnancy, your Miracle Journey is walked alone. What a wonderful revelation that can become! You have this precious time when you alone commune with your child. Through imagination, take your baby's hand and walk together. Glory in the simplicity of solitude. All too soon it will come to an end, and you will give birth, presenting your child to the world.

I watch, and am as a sparrow alone upon the house top.
—Psalm 102:7, KJV

Day 1

These are only a shadow of what is to come, but the substance belongs to Christ. *Colossians 2:17*

_____

_____

_____

Day 2

For God alone my soul waits in silence, for my hope is from him. *Psalm 62:5*

_____

_____

_____

Day 3

Look on my right hand and see—there is no one who takes notice of me; no refuge remains to me; no one cares for me. I cry to you, O Lord; I say, "You are my refuge, my portion in the land of the living." *Psalm 142:4-5*

_____

_____

_____

Day 4

God, the Lord, is my strength; he makes my feet like the feet of a deer, and makes me tread upon the heights. *Habakkuk 3:19*

_____

_____

_____

Day 5

Be careful then how you live, not as unwise people but as wise, making the most of the time, because the days are evil. So do not be foolish, but understand what the will of the Lord is. *Ephesians 5:15-17*

_____

_____

Day 6

The widow who is really in need and left all alone puts her hope in God and continues night and day to pray and to ask God for help. *1 Timothy 5:5, NIV*

_____

_____

Day 7

You are worthy, our Lord and God, to receive glory and honor and power, for you created all things, and by your will they existed and were created. *Revelation 4:11*

_____

_____

35

Third Month

Weeks 13~16

Prayer for the Child

Lord, your miracle is now four inches long and weighs over one ounce. Your hand has touched fingers and toes, giving them soft, delicate nails. Lord, you indeed are all knowing, for even now you plan for the future of our child by secretly tucking away twenty buds for baby teeth. Delicate hair is beginning to appear on our child's precious head. I imagine your loving hand stroking the first tiny locks, for you already know their very number. I stand in amazement that with a simple command, you've told the kidneys to get to work, giving the go-ahead for the processing of fluids within such an immature system. O gracious Creator, bless all the organs that are now formed and will continue to develop and mature. Nurture this precious seed, and prepare its soul to accept your gift of salvation. Make our child perfect and whole, a glorious example of your magnificence. Amen.

Prayer for the Mother

Thank you, Lord, for teaching me how to cope with all the physical side effects of this Miracle Journey. I'm learning patience and endurance as I take one day at a time. I have a new sense of calmness and peace. That is probably because I've started unbuttoning my waistbands. I'm beginning to see the first subtle signs of a blossoming new me. Help me to like this new me, this new body. Let me choose joy in accepting my maternal self with laughter. O, my brilliant Creator, I'm loving you with a new sense of wonder as this startling gift grows inside of me. Thank you for the husband you gave to me, and the miracle of two becoming one. Bless the man whose precious love now resides within me, in our child. Prepare the waiting family for this unfolding miracle: the baby's brothers and sisters, the grandparents, the aunts and uncles, and the cousins. Thank you for their interest and encouragement. Amen.

Theme of the month: Love

God's love is surrounding you today and always. Inside you is your child—a child you will love like no other person in your life. The Miracle Journey is a time of preparing for the unimaginable love of motherhood. If you are not feeling very loving or lovable, ask God to help you clothe yourself in love (Colossians 3:14). Your heavenly Father will be faithful and send the Holy Spirit to help you do that. Feed your soul with words of love. Memorize a favorite verse to meditate on as you learn to embrace love each day.

Bible Study

Read the Song of Solomon. Then write a love letter to your husband and to your unborn child.

May your love for
each other help
awaken
The world that the
world longs to be,
For, as poetry is the
undying language
of love,
Love is the undying
poetry of being.
—Kate Farrell

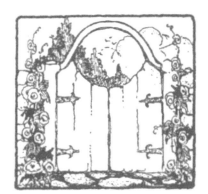

*P*ERHAPS you've been blessed by seeing a black-and-white vision of your baby in the sonogram. It's truly miraculous to see the four chambers of the heart beating. How delightful to watch as your child kicks and squirms, turns and dances within your womb! You might discover your child's gender, watch the fetus suck its thumb, or see a skeletal impression of the baby's future face. Lennart Nilsson wrote an incredible book, *A Child Is Born*. On these pages are actual photographs of the fetus from conception through birth, giving us an interior view of the Miracle Journey.

At this stage in your journey, you may be faced with the decision of whether to undergo prenatal testing. Your doctor alone should not decide whether you will have prenatal tests. You and your husband should make those decisions after discussing the pros and cons with your doctor. If you are torn with indecision, pray for wisdom and seek wise counsel from your medical provider, friends, other pregnant women who have undergone prenatal testing, or your pastor. Most important, talk honestly with your mate about what the results will mean to you.

Types of Prenatal Tests

Ultrasound (sonogram) is performed at any stage of pregnancy. Ultrasound creates an image of the fetus from sound waves. It can provide valuable information about the fetus's health, such as age of the fetus, rate of growth, placement of the placenta, amount of amniotic fluid in the uterus, fetal position, movement, breathing, heart rate, possibly gender, number of fetuses, and some birth defects. No harmful effects to either the mother or the baby have been found in over twenty years of use.

Chorionic villus sampling (CVS) is performed between weeks 8 and 12. Results can be obtained within ten days, allowing a diagnosis to be made before the end of the first trimester. The procedure involves inserting a catheter through the vagina and cervix into the placenta. Chorionic villi cells (microscopic, finger-like projections that make up the placenta) are withdrawn and grown in a special culture; then their genetic makeup is analyzed. Most common risk associated with CVS is miscarriage (increased by 1 to 3 percent when CVS is performed).

Amniocentesis is performed between weeks 14 and 18 or even as late as week 20. It can take two to four weeks to analyze the results. The procedure involves inserting a needle through the abdomen into the uterus and amniotic sac. Fluid is withdrawn, grown in a special culture, and analyzed, based on your personal and family medical history. Occasional side effects include cramping, vaginal bleeding, and leaking of amniotic fluid. Injury to fetus is rare, and miscarriage is increased by only 0.5 percent.

Alpha-fetoprotein (AFP) is performed between weeks 15 and 18, but can be performed as late as week 20. Results can be obtained within ten days. AFP is a simple blood test that measures the amount of a chemical called alpha-fetoprotein in the mother's blood. This test helps identify women who might be carrying a fetus with a neural tube defect. If this disorder is present, knowing your baby has a neural tube defect will help doctors manage a safer delivery for your baby.

Day 1

Whenever you face trials of any kind, consider it nothing but joy, because you know that the testing of your faith produces endurance. *James 1:2-3*

_____

_____

Day 2

My frame was not hidden from you, when I was being made in secret, intricately woven in the depths of the earth. Your eyes beheld my unformed substance. In your book were written all the days that were formed for me, when none of them as yet existed. *Psalm 139:15-16*

_____

_____

Day 3

Every good and perfect gift is from above, coming down from the Father of the heavenly lights, who does not change like shifting shadows. He chose to give us birth through the word of truth, that we might be a kind of firstfruits of all he created. *James 1:17-18, NIV*

_____

_____

Day 4

You hem me in, behind and before, and lay your hand upon me. *Psalm 139:5*

_____

_____

Day 5

The heavens declare the glory of God; the skies proclaim the work of his hands. *Psalm 19:1, NIV*

_____

_____

Day 6

Ever since the creation of the world his eternal power and divine nature, invisible though they are, have been understood and seen through the things he has made. So they are without excuse. *Romans 1:20*

_____

_____

Day 7

The wisdom from above is first pure, then peaceable, gentle, willing to yield, full of mercy and good fruits, without a trace of partiality or hypocrisy. *James 3:17*

_____

_____

_____

W E'VE all heard of mothers who played music to their wombs, classical, jazz, or lullabies that vibrate through the bodily walls and drift into the unborn's ears. After the child is born, those same melodies seem to calm the cries from colic and soothe the newborn into a peaceful sleep. How much more important than music are the prayers of a mother's heart for her child's lifetime? What are your hopes for your baby? Maybe your hopes include health, opportunity, peace, and joy. You might want to cultivate character traits such as courage, honesty, respect, and loyalty.

Think about what's most important for this child and list the top three hopes and character traits.

Top three hopes	Top three character traits
_____	_____
_____	_____
_____	_____

We can parent to produce character traits by teaching, discipline, and modeling the traits we deem important. But a mother can only pray for her hopes, for your hopes are out of your hands, fulfilled only by the sovereign God. When you set goals for your child's character traits, you help to prioritize the limits you set and the discipline tactics you use. Thus you work toward effective parenting.

A mother of four told me that a mother's prayer radiates to heaven like a beacon of light. Many times I've frantically prayed, "Lord, help!" God has always answered that distress call.

Melodee M. Young lists twelve things a mother should pray for her children:

That your child will develop a thankful and generous heart and a positive attitude.
That your child will mature, increasing mentally, physically, spiritually, and socially.
That your child will develop a strong sense of family love and unity and keep vows.
That your child will seek a relationship with God and have a deep desire to do his will.
That your child will develop a love for God's Word and learn to apply it to decision making.
That your child will hate evil and cling to what is good, taking a stand for Christ.
That God will protect your child from evil and all Satan's trickery in every area of life.
That God will enable your child to overcome temptations to sin and avoid sinful habits.
That nothing will hinder your maturing child from accepting Christ as Savior and Lord.
That God will reveal the work he has planned for your child,
and that your child will be successful and satisfied with it.
That your child will be blessed with godly mentors and will respect and submit to proper authorities.
That your child's life will be a witness to the hope, love, and saving power of Christ.

Commit yourself to praying for each of the twelve areas. A good way to do this is to designate one area to each calendar month and then enhance the topic as it fits the needs of your child.

The greatest gift I can give my children is to be their prayer warrior.
—Melodee M. Young

A mother's prayers are a beacon of light to the Father God.

Day 1

Let your ear now be attentive, and your eyes open, that you may hear the prayer of your servant, which I pray before you now, day and night, for the children. *Nehemiah 1:6, KJV, adapted*

_____

_____

_____

Day 2

Let my prayer be counted as incense before you, and the lifting up of my hands as an evening sacrifice. *Psalm 141:2*

_____

_____

_____

Day 3

Rejoice in hope, be patient in suffering, persevere in prayer. *Romans 12:12*

_____

_____

_____

Day 4

Continue in prayer, and watch in the same with thanksgiving. *Colossians 4:2, KJV*

_____

_____

_____

Day 5

Rejoice always, pray without ceasing, give thanks in all circumstances; for this is the will of God in Christ Jesus for you. *1 Thessalonians 5:16-18*

_____

_____

_____

Day 6

Do not worry about anything, but in everything by prayer and supplication with thanksgiving let your requests be made known to God. *Philippians 4:6*

_____

_____

_____

Day 7

For this child I prayed; and the Lord has granted me the petition that I made to him. Therefore I have lent him to the Lord; as long as he lives, he is given to the Lord. *1 Samuel 1:27-28*

_____

_____

Because my first child, Morgen, was born at twenty-four weeks and died six months later,
my second pregnancy was filled with anxiety. I was "high risk"
and lived at the doctor's office.
Although every sonogram (at least eight) and every prenatal test (I had them all)
showed that I was having a normal pregnancy and a healthy baby,
I still had that nagging thought that something bad was going to happen.
All my fears vanished when I heard my beautiful baby boy, Garrett, cry for the first time.
It was the sound of victory after a long battle.
—Becky D. Hayslip

YOUR Miracle Journey could be a treacherous battle, every step taken with trepidation and bountiful prayers. You want so much—and yet you may bury your hope, love, and excitement, especially if your route has been labeled "high risk."

Being pregnant is suddenly the most vulnerable experience you have had to endure. You begin to understand the risks involved even in "normal" pregnancies and child rearing. You have opened yourself up to more second-guessing, fear, and heartache than you have ever experienced in your life. The mere thought of anything going wrong or endangering your precious baby makes you shudder with fear and tense with protectiveness.

Nevertheless, this is what it means to be a mother: to protect with a dimension that transcends your vulnerability and fear because you love your child so deeply. The Creator has given you a mother's love, so tenacious and proverbial for people and animals.

This need to protect your child is an instinctive urge that begins before the baby leaves the womb. When confronted with danger, other humans protect their faces, but a pregnant woman will protect her stomach. This fierce drive to defend your baby makes you stronger than you ever thought you could be. To care for your child, you are prepared to do anything, withstand anything, and sacrifice anything as you stand on your faith in God. Blessedly, your husband is also part of the protective fence that God has placed around you and the baby.

Your love becomes a shield of faith, strengthened with hope, fortified with prayers, and made steadfast with all the extra care you and your husband must take against the *risks* set before you. You wrap this shield of love around your baby, ready to fight the battles ahead to keep your child safe.

When you are faced with the unthinkable, believe the unbelievable.

Oh, what a power is motherhood, possessing a potent spell.
All mothers alike fight fiercely for a child.
—Euripides

Day 1

Have you not put a hedge around Job and his household and everything he has? You have blessed the work of his hands, so that his flocks and herds are spread throughout the land. *Job 1:10, NIV, adapted.* Pray that God will build a hedge of protection around you and your child.

_____

_____

Day 2

You hem me in, behind and before, and lay your hand upon me. *Psalm 139:5*

_____

_____

Day 3

But let all who take refuge in you rejoice; let them ever sing for joy. Spread your protection over them, so that those who love your name may exult in you. *Psalm 5:11*

_____

_____

Day 4

God has not given us the spirit of fear; but of power, and of love, and of a sound mind. *2 Timothy 1:7, KJV, adapted*

_____

_____

Day 5

Take action, for it is your duty, and we are with you; be strong, and do it. *Ezra 10:4*

_____

_____

Day 6

Christ is faithful as a son over God's house. And we are his house, if we hold on to our courage and the hope of which we boast. *Hebrews 3:6, NIV*

_____

_____

Day 7

Be strong and bold; have no fear or dread of them, because it is the Lord your God who goes with you; he will not fail you or forsake you. *Deuteronomy 31:6*

_____

_____

PREGNANCY and all its surrounding glory changes more than just your swelling waistline, bustline, and ankles. You might feel like an alien has taken over your personality; you become a stranger even to yourself, with out-of-this-world behavior.

You ride a pendulum that often swings from one extreme emotion to the other in a single heartbeat. Joy turns to tears. Anger to uncontrollable giggles. Frustration to contentment. You are at times unpredictable and inconsolable. In real life, your family sees something of a Dr. Jekyll and Mr. Hyde personality played out in mind-boggling scenes.

During my first pregnancy, my husband was unprepared for this radical change in my easygoing, dependable personality. He had no idea how to handle my weepy, fall-to-pieces, delicate-as-china, and moody-as-a-mad-monkey psyche. I wasn't always reasonable, and he simply didn't know how to deal with my out-of-whack emotions.

Michael pampered, placated, and pacified me. No matter what I asked, he answered, "Whatever you want, darling." Then he walked away, shaking his head, when his best efforts were met with near hysteria. I complained, "Unless you have a uterus, you can't understand." By month 5, my extremely frustrated husband had lost all sympathy. Michael wanted me to "snap out of it" and insisted that my obstetrician could do "something" to get my emotions in balance. He wanted me fixed and back to normal. However, hormones don't listen to logic, and the mate tends to become frustrated.

Therefore, fortify yourself with the understanding that pregnant women at times aren't easy to live with. Become sensitized to your changing moods. Empower yourself with self-control. Take special care not to exploit and rationalize your unpredictable behavior. Don't use your hormones as an excuse for being a shrew.

Although the expectant father might not be experiencing sympathy pregnancy pains, have some sympathy for *his* unique Miracle Journey. Amidst all the joy, excitement, and discovery, a future father may think that the Miracle Journey is a trial. At times he wonders if he's ever going to get his "old" reliable wife back. Never fear! This too shall pass—but not to become exactly what was before. The father too will be forever changed by the birth of that baby, and so will your marriage relationship and your enlarged family. You are companions on a journey, and God's Spirit is your guide.

The fruit of the Spirit is
love, joy, peace,
patience, kindness, generosity, faithfulness,
gentleness, and self-control.
—Galatians 5:22-23

Lord, empower me with your Holy Spirit. Let me choose self-control, joy, peace, patience, kindness, generosity, faithfulness, gentleness, and love—especially to my beloved mate. Amen.

Who are you?
And what have you
done with my wife?
—Michael Kelly

Day 1

Like a city breached, without walls, is one who lacks self-control. *Proverbs 25:28*

_____

_____

_____

Day 2

From the same mouth come blessing and cursing. My brothers and sisters, this ought not to be so. *James 3:10*

_____

_____

_____

Day 3

If they desire life and desire to see good days, let them keep their tongues from evil and their lips from speaking deceit; let them turn away from evil and do good; let them seek peace and pursue it. *1 Peter 3:10-11, adapted*

_____

_____

Day 4

Sing praises to the Lord, O you his faithful ones, and give thanks to his holy name. For his anger is but for a moment; his favor is for a lifetime. Weeping may linger for the night, but joy comes with the morning. *Psalm 30:4-5*

_____

_____

Day 5

It is better to live in a desert land than with a contentious and fretful spouse. *Proverbs 21:19, adapted*

_____

_____

_____

Day 6

A quarrelsome spouse is like a constant dripping. *Proverbs 19:13, NIV, adapted*

_____

_____

_____

Day 7

It is better to dwell in a corner of the house top, than with a brawling spouse in a wide house. *Proverbs 21:9, KJV, adapted*

_____

_____

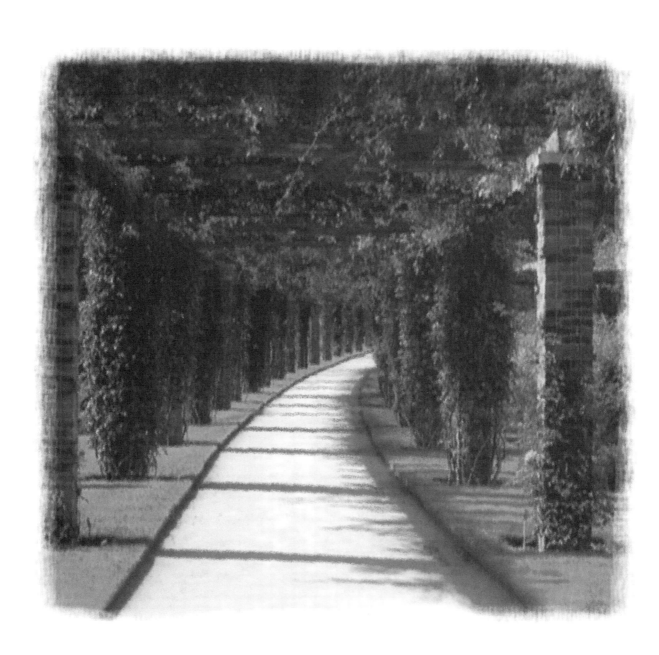

The Second Trimester

Being Prepared

It's time to reorganize your closet. As your waist increases, your usable wardrobe decreases. Move unwearable items to the back of the closet; arrange your maternity clothes in the front.

Decide where you will set up the nursery. Start pricing the essentials, and research baby products for safety and consumer satisfaction. When it comes to buying for your baby, be an educated consumer.

As questions arise, write them down to discuss with your doctor.

Research what's ahead for you and your baby in the next three months.

Planning and Doing

Are you preparing your children for the arrival of a new brother or sister?

Are you investigating childcare? Are you putting your name on waiting lists and looking at options?

Have you decided on the length of your maternity leave? Are you setting money aside to compensate for the income lost during an extended leave? Are you leaving paper trails at work? Are you preparing co-workers for your absence?

Have you picked a destination for a last-fling getaway for yourselves as parents-to-be? This middle trimester will be the best time for a vacation.

Goal-Setting

Confirm the lifestyle changes you vowed on week 5.

How's your weight gain? Are you meeting your exercise goals and eating healthful foods?

Are you staying on budget? Are you saving for the things you deemed important?

Keeping a Journal

Commit yourself to recording your journey daily. Don't just write down what you ate, how long you walked, and how much you slept. Chronicle your feelings, body changes, fears, excitement, and daily dilemmas. Write down the funny, touching, or thought-provoking things people say. Are you having crazy dreams? Do you crave weird foods? Are you meeting new pregnant friends? Have you bought new maternity outfits?

Don't forget to take photographs of your changing body. You'll see a vast transformation in the next three months.

Fourth Month

Weeks 17~20

Prayer for the Child

Inside me, O Master Planner, you've created the perfect playground for our tiny one. The babe-in-the-womb now moves, somersaults, kicks, sleeps, and wakes at intervals. You've taught the wee one to swallow and to pass urine as our child's system begins the never-ending cycle of processing fluids. I delight in the knowledge that our baby can already hear our voices and express emotions with new-formed eyebrows. The precious skin is transparent and pink. I smile with joy because our child is now as long as my hand and weighs five ounces. Bless each new development, that it will be as perfect as you designed it to be. Amen.

Prayer for the Mother

O gracious Lord, my joy is so great. Finally I can feel the lightest flutterings inside of me. Your little one feels like a playful butterfly, and in rare moments you include me in the frolicking fun. I glow with my delight. This miracle is starting to feel real. I'm even starting to almost look pregnant. I thank you for my renewed strength and energy. Help me to accept the changes occurring in my appearance, and remind me they are only temporary. Let me chose joy each morning when I awake, ever thankful that you have given us a miracle. Thank you for letting me feel this precious child, and let each flutter renew my love for you. Amen.

Rejoice!

This month is full of changes. You will probably shed some of the unpleasant symptoms of pregnancy and feel renewed by the new growth from within. You're on the verge of really *feeling* pregnant, and your precious cargo is ready to introduce itself to you as you move through a new stage of the Miracle Journey.

Rejuvenate! Rejoice! You have new energy and a new realization of your destination.

Write a few lines of a favorite hymn, psalm, or song. Meditate on the passage.

Make a joyful noise to the Lord, all the earth.
Worship the Lord with gladness; come into his presence with singing.
Know that the Lord is God. It is he that made us, and we are his;
we are his people, and the sheep of his pasture.
Enter his gates with thanksgiving, and his courts with praise.
Give thanks to him, bless his name.
For the Lord is good; his steadfast love endures forever,
and his faithfulness to all generations.
—Psalm 100

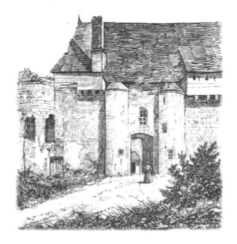

My husband was gone on a business trip for a week.
On the night he returned, he walked in on me preparing for bed.
"Oh, my!" He stared open-mouthed at my bare, bulging belly. "You're huge!"
"I'm what?" I lifted a brow in caution.
"You're huge, in a great way, not a big way,"
he quickly explained as he touched my belly.
"Wow, I can finally see the baby!"
—Martha Robuck

JUST when you learn to adjust to the rigors of morning sickness and fatigue, they mysteriously go away. What fit you yesterday, doesn't fit today. You stand in the middle of your closet with absolutely nothing to wear. You watch your belly grow bigger with each passing breath. No doubt, the minute you've accepted your new body shape, voilà, it changes again, and your rounding belly catches someone by surprise.

I remember the most traumatic body-changing moment of my first pregnancy. I had gone on a three-mile walk. I went upstairs to shower and change. As I peeled down the bike shorts, I went into emotional shock. My waist had disappeared! My pear-shaped body had always had a small pinched-in waist; suddenly, that asset was gone. *Gone*, I tell you. In one hour of exercise, I had lost my waist and my prepregnancy figure.

Immediately I called my best friend as I stood gaping at the mirror in disbelief. "I lost my waist!" I cried in horror. Debbie, a new mother, casually sighed, "Just wait till you lose your belly button." Visualizing the impossible, as I looked at my still-flat stomach, I gulped, "Belly button?" Debbie's laughter eased, and she gently encouraged me, "Jess, it's okay. You'll lose a few things along the way, but your body does go back to normal. I promise."

Learning to accept yourself in a new and expanding body is hard at first. Your stunned spouse might not be the best source for assurance that everything will come out in the wash. Find women who have finished the Miracle Journey; they will encourage you. Keep reminding yourself that your expanded body is only a temporary condition. During your pregnancy, you will constantly need to adjust to change. Even if you are not quite the same after pregnancy as before, it's not the end of the world.

It's important to remember that all this change is not just physical change. You're adjusting to changing feelings and emotions. You're forging a new relationship with your mate as you bring a child into your family. You're learning to give up some of your independence as you prepare to share yourself with a child. You're in transit to a new identity called motherhood.

Remember that the Miracle Journey is a passage of transformation. Thank God that he gives us forty weeks to slowly go through several stages of change, preparing us to accept the miracle of our baby.

Let us consider how to provoke one another to love and good deeds, not neglecting to meet together, as is the habit of some, but encouraging one another, and all the more as you see the Day approaching.
—Hebrews 10:24-25

Day 1

You are my hiding place and my shield; I hope in your word. *Psalm 119:114*

_____

_____

_____

Day 2

Do not be conformed to this world, but be transformed by the renewing of your minds, so that you may discern what is the will of God—what is good and acceptable and perfect. *Romans 12:2*

_____

Day 3

Restore us to yourself, O Lord, that we may be restored; renew our days as of old. *Lamentations 5:21*

_____

_____

_____

Day 4

Create in me a clean heart, O God, and put a new and right spirit within me. *Psalm 51:10*

_____

_____

Day 5

The Lord Jesus Christ . . . , by his power to rule all things, . . . will change our simple bodies and make them like his own glorious body. *Philippians 3:20-21, NCV*

_____

_____

Day 6

Isaac went out in the evening to walk in the field. *Genesis 24:63*
Run to win! . . . Use self-control. . . . I do not run without a goal. I treat my body hard and make it my slave. *1 Corinthians 9:25-27, NCV*

_____

_____

Day 7

Train yourself in godliness, for, while physical training is of some value, godliness is valuable in every way, holding promise for both the present life and the life to come. *1 Timothy 4:7-8*

_____

_____

Pop quiz: Did you exercise today? Did you work out with your body and your mind in preparing and planning for your child, and with your spirit in meditation and prayer?

_____

_____

YOU'VE unbuttoned waistbands, eased down zippers, and worn the same skirt three times this week. Let's face it: your nonexistent waist and thickening tummy are suffering in your old wardrobe. You don't look so great when you try to squeeze into regular-size clothes, and you feel restricted and uncomfortable. You also might split some seams. So it's time to move into the world of *maternity clothes*.

Unless you have unlimited funds, *think* before you run out and buy a whole new wardrobe. Maternity clothes tend to be expensive, and you wear them for a short time. You want to stretch your money.

How to Build a Smart Maternity Wardrobe

Spend a few hours reorganizing your closet. Look at every item you own and evaluate it. Have you worn this in the past two years? If not, cut the emotional strings and put it in a box for a consignment store or for charity. If yes, can you wear this item in the months ahead? If not, reject it. Pull aside anything expandable that can still be worn comfortably.

Now move the rejects to the back of your closet and use the space in front for maternity clothes. What do you have to work with from your existing wardrobe? Maybe you don't have much, but don't panic. Begin building your wardrobe by making some phone calls to friends and family. Ask where they shopped for their maternity wardrobe and if you may *borrow*. (Keep a list of what you borrow from whom, or write their name in permanent marker on the tags.)

After you have collected clothes on loan from others, look at what you have. Bottoms are the key component. Do you have skirts and slacks in basic solid colors? If your job dictates that you must dress for success, do you have career pieces? What are your needs, based on your lifestyle? Make a wish list and prioritize it. Decide on a first-shopping-trip budget. Then let your fingers do the walking through the Yellow Pages before you set out. Is there a resale maternity shop in your area? What department stores carry maternity clothes? Make a list of maternity specialty stores. Don't forget discount stores; they're usually a gold mine of basics. Women's clothes in large sizes can be great substitutes for maternity items, so check out those departments as well.

Fashion Hints for Downsizing an Expanding Belly

Dark colors, vertical stripes, small prints, and solid colors worn head-to-toe are most slenderizing.

Don't accentuate your waist; you don't have one! *Don't* tuck in. That is a maternity no-no.

Layers camouflage. Vests and loose jackets are terrific. A man's shirt can look great when paired with leggings or worn as a jacket.

To get the most from your wardrobe, buy basics first and build up. Remember that you can mix separates and wear them several ways, especially if you keep your wardrobe in interchangeable color families that work together: black, white, red, navy.

Don't try to hide your pregnancy! Why would you want to do that? Pregnancy is a delight, not a disgrace! Your goal is to be pregnant and attractive at the same time.

"I love being pregnant, and that joyful attitude makes me glow." Then she whispered, *"Of course, dressing the part helps. It's truly all in the packaging."* —Barbie Johnson Reilly

52

Strength and dignity are her clothing, and she smiles at the future. —Proverbs 31:25, NAS

Day 1

For the Lord does not see as mortals see; they look on the outward appearance, but the Lord looks on the heart. *1 Samuel 16:7*

Day 2

I will greatly rejoice in the Lord, my whole being shall exult in my God; for he has clothed me with the garments of salvation, he has covered me with the robe of righteousness, as a bridegroom decks himself with a garland, and as a bride adorns herself with her jewels. *Isaiah 61:10*

Day 3

The angel said to those who were standing before him, "Take off his filthy clothes." And to him he said, "See, I have taken your guilt away from you, and I will clothe you with festal apparel." *Zechariah 3:4*

Day 4

Bestow on them a crown of beauty instead of ashes, the oil of gladness instead of mourning, and a garment of praise instead of a spirit of despair. *Isaiah 61:3, NIV*

55

Day 5

You have stripped off the old self with its practices and have clothed yourselves with the new self, which is being renewed in knowledge according to the image of its creator. *Colossians 3:9-10*

Day 6

Heaven and earth will perish, but you remain; they will all wear out like clothing; like a cloak you will roll them up, and like clothing they will be changed. But you are the same, and your years will never end. *Hebrews 1:11-12, adapted*

Day 7

I put on righteousness, and it clothed me; my justice was like a robe and a turban. *Job 29:14*

Being pregnant is like walking around with a sign that says,
ADVICE WANTED.
—Debbie Boyd

*I*T'S inevitable: when a person finds out you are pregnant, regardless of whether that person has a uterus or has ever been pregnant, she or he immediately starts giving advice. These impromptu counseling sessions can happen anywhere. The grocery line, a crowded elevator, or even a formal business meeting can turn into a no-holds-barred debate on the pros and cons of natural delivery.

Strangers who would probably never say hello will assume that it's okay to reach out and touch your belly. People will astound you with their "wealth" of information and old wives' tales. Strangers will offend and shock you with their forthrightness and criticism. Some well-meaning advice-giver will ultimately scare you speechless with a tragic or horrific story!

I quickly caught on to the advice game. The opening question of "When are you due, dear?" is really the prelude for giving a pregnant woman unwanted advice. I learned to put filters on my ears and set boundaries for my intake of advice.

Always consider the source. Do these people *know* what they're talking about? Did they have children? How old are their children? A lot has changed in obstetrics in the past five years alone, not to speak of twenty-five years!

Next, if you know the advice-givers personally, look at their lives. Do these advisors practice what they preach, talk the talk, or walk the walk? Are they justified in telling you that you eat too much sodium when their ankles are bigger than yours? Where did their level of expertise come from?

Finally, try my way around unwanted advice. I directed it to something I didn't mind talking about. When the inevitable question was asked, I answered, "I'm due on November 15. We're having the hardest time coming up with names. How did you find a name for your child?" Another possibility: "I'm searching for a good pediatrician. Do you know one in the area?" Asking broad, open-ended, direct questions can keep a conversation from going into dangerous, spooky, unwanted waters—even when talking with the stranger in the grocery line.

Therefore, sift advice like wheat, to separate the seed from the chaff. I would have never made it through the Miracle Journey without the mothers who had already walked it ahead of me. They bolstered, cheered, and encouraged me through every step. Advice from the right source is a godsend. When you reach a rocky path or stand amidst a raging storm in your Miracle Journey, seek out a wise counselor.

Beloved, do not believe every spirit, but test the spirits to see whether they are from God;
for many false prophets have gone out into the world. . . .
Little children, you are from God, and have conquered them;
for the one who is in you is greater than the one who is in the world.
—1 John 4:1, 4

Day 1

Fools think their own way is right, but the wise listen to advice. *Proverbs 12:15*

_____

_____

_____

Day 2

Where there is no guidance, a nation falls, but in an abundance of counselors there is safety. *Proverbs 11:14*

_____

_____

_____

Day 3

David said to Abigail, "Blessed be the Lord, the God of Israel, who sent you to meet me today! Blessed be your good sense, and blessed be you, who have kept me today from bloodguilt and from avenging myself by my own hand!" *1 Samuel 25:32-33*

_____

_____

Day 4

Therefore encourage one another and build up each other, as indeed you are doing. *1 Thessalonians 5:11*

_____

_____

_____

Day 5

Is wisdom with the aged, and understanding in length of days? "With God are wisdom and strength; he has counsel and understanding." *Job 12:12-13*

_____

_____

_____

Day 6

I, wisdom from God, have good advice and sound wisdom; I have insight, I have strength. *Proverbs 8:14, adapted*

_____

_____

_____

Day 7

The purposes in the human mind are like deep water, but the intelligent will draw them out. *Proverbs 20:5*

_____

_____

_____

Jesus said to his disciples, "Therefore I tell you, do not worry about your life,
what you will eat, or about your body, what you will wear.
For life is more than food, and the body more than clothing.
Consider the ravens: they neither sow nor reap, they have neither storehouse nor barn,
and yet God feeds them. Of how much more value are you than the birds!
And can any of you by worrying add a single hour to your span of life?
If then you are not able to do so small a thing as that, why do you worry about the rest?
Consider the lilies, how they grow: they neither toil nor spin;
yet I tell you, even Solomon in all his glory was not clothed like one of these.
But if God so clothes the grass of the field, which is alive today and tomorrow is thrown into
the oven, how much more will he clothe you—you of little faith!
And do not keep striving for what you are to eat and what you are to drink,
and do not keep worrying. For it is the nations of the world that strive after all these things,
and your Father knows that you need them.
Instead, strive for his kingdom, and these things will be given to you as well.
Do not be afraid, little flock, for it is your Father's good pleasure to give you the kingdom."
—Luke 12:22-31

Paste here a
photograph
of yourself,
at week 20.
You're
halfway
there!

You Are Beautiful!

Today, _____, I am halfway through the Miracle Journey.
Up to this point, most of the changes have occurred inside my body.
Now our beloved child is busy growing, moving, and playing.
My body is re-forming to accommodate this ever-changing miracle.

Day 1

For who is God except the Lord? And who is a rock besides our God?—the God who girded me with strength, and made my way safe. He made my feet like the feet of a deer, and set me secure on the heights. *Psalm 18:31-33*

_____

_____

Day 2

My dove, my perfect one, is the only one, the darling of her mother, flawless to her that bore her. *Song of Solomon 6:9*

_____

_____

Day 3

A cheerful heart is a good medicine, but a downcast spirit dries up the bones. *Proverbs 17:22*

_____

_____

Day 4

Take heed now, for the Lord has chosen you to build a house as the sanctuary; be strong, and act. *1 Chronicles 28:10*

_____

_____

57

Day 5

"Come," my heart says, "seek his face!" Your face, Lord, do I seek. *Psalm 27:8*

_____

_____

Day 6

It shall blossom abundantly, and rejoice even with joy and singing. *Isaiah 35:2, KJV*

_____

_____

Day 7

Let the peace of Christ rule in your hearts. . . . And be thankful. *Colossians 3:15*

_____

_____

Pop quiz: List five things for which you are grateful today.

_____

_____

_____

_____

Fifth Month

Weeks 21~24

Prayer for the Child

O Lord, although our child is but a cocooned fetus that weighs less than a pound and is only eight to twelve inches long, you've already established order and gifted this child with an innate schedule of activity. How wondrous it is to me that our tiny child now sleeps and wakes in regular intervals. Our baby turns, rolls, kicks, and stretches. Lord, give our child all the things it needs through my obedience to healthful eating, exercise, stress reduction, and rest. I know the internal organs are still maturing, and they need my help to make them healthy. It's hard to believe this little one's fingernails have grown to the tips of tiny fingers. Bless our child with developing creativity to praise your holy name through art, music, or words. Pour out your strength upon this child. Guide our child's path until this miracle of yours is placed into our waiting arms of love. Amen.

Prayer for the Mother

I think I'm going crazy, Lord. My thoughts are often scattered to the wind, and I've never been so forgetful or absentminded. Nothing seems to be working right, including my interior plumbing. But I know you're the Master Plumber. You designed my system for the Miracle Journey. So help me to do my part in this short process. Let me eat right. Let me reach for water, lots of water, when I'd rather have that soda or coffee. Give me an appetite for the things this child needs, not the empty foods I know aren't worth the calories. Remind me that the discomforts of pregnancy are temporary. Lord, thank you for the passage of time; I can feel the "cargo" I'm carrying now. I delight in the baby's kicks and other movements you've let me share. May they always bring a smile amidst the discomforts I'm suffering. Amen.

Get Away from It All

This is the month to plan a special getaway. You're feeling better, and you both deserve it. Whether you can afford a week, weekend, or only an overnight trip, just do it! Get away, relax, and enjoy time alone with your mate. Take a holiday now. Five months from now, it won't be so simple to pack up and go. There already is a lot going on in your life. When Jesus and his disciples were too busy, he said, "Come away to a deserted place all by yourselves and rest a while" (Mark 6:31). Follow the great Master's advice.

Our Getaway Vacation Plans

_____

_____

_____

_____

_____

_____

_____

_____

_____

_____

_____

_____

_____

_____

_____

_____

_____

_____

_____

_____

_____

_____

_____

My daughter, shall I not seek rest for you, that it may be well with you?
—Ruth 3:1, KJV, adapted

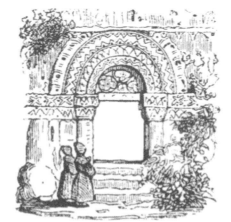

"Move over!" said the uterus to the bladder,
which bumped the kidney, which jostled the pelvis, which spread the hips,
which stretched the ligaments,
which made the back ache, weighed down the shoulders, and shortened the breath.

YOU'RE feeling a twitch at the waist and a tightness in your groin. You're lower back is aching, or your shoulders thud with a nagging pang. There might even be a sharp, piercing pain that throws your eyebrows to your hairline and sends you running for the phone to call your doctor.

Go ahead and make that call. At this stage of the journey, no matter how many times you've experienced pregnancy before, you're likely to have a list of unusual aches and pains and uneasy feelings about what's really going on inside your changing body.

The most common growing pain, characteristic during weeks 18 to 24, is groin or abdominal hurting. As the baby grows, the bands of fibrous tissue, or round ligaments, along both sides of the uterus are pulled and stretched to support the increasing size of the uterus. You may feel this as sharp pains in your abdomen (usually on the sides) or a dull, nagging ache. Round-ligament pain is often most noticeable when you rise too quickly from a chair or bed or when you cough or sneeze.

It's hard to believe that up until week 12 of gestation, your entire uterus was able to fit inside your pelvis. By week 20, the top of your uterus has reached your navel. Now your womb's globular bulk starts to nudge other interior organs out of its way, and your thickened waist begins to extend outward. During this intense growth stage of the journey, your body must reorganize and adjust. Thus, you have entered the twilight zone of weird and unusual growing pains.

It is written,
"No eye has seen, nor ear heard,
nor the human heart conceived,
what God has prepared for those who love him."
—1 Corinthians 2:9, adapted

Day 1

For in hope we were saved. Now hope that is seen is not hope. For who hopes for what is seen? But if we hope for what we do not see, we wait for it with patience. *Romans 8:24-25*

_____

_____

Day 2

It is good to give thanks to the Lord, to sing praises to your name, O Most High; to declare your steadfast love in the morning, and your faithfulness by night. *Psalm 92:1-2*

_____

_____

Day 3

Who knows? Perhaps you have come to royal dignity for just such a time as this. *Esther 4:14*

_____

_____

_____

Day 4

Neither the one who plants nor the one who waters is anything, but only God who gives the growth. *1 Corinthians 3:7*

_____

_____

Day 5

Grow in the grace and knowledge of our Lord and Savior Jesus Christ. To him be the glory both now and to the day of eternity. Amen. *2 Peter 3:18*

_____

_____

Day 6

O Lord, all my longing is known to you; my sighing is not hidden from you. *Psalm 38:9*

_____

_____

_____

Day 7

Mary got up and went quickly to a town in the hills of Judea. She came to Zechariah's house and greeted Elizabeth. *Luke 1:39-40*

_____

_____

Pop quiz: Are you planning your getaway vacation? You need it, and more important, you and your mate deserve it.

_____

_____

61

Ah! Here, right here, hurry! Put your hand here.
Now wait, be patient, wait. . . . Did you feel it?
—Laurie McClure

NOT long ago you desperately wanted to feel the first kick. You questioned that first delicate flutter—uncertain, wondering, marveling as your child came to life through movements. Now you are regularly reminded of your baby's presence, kicking, twirling, and dancing within your body, leaping for joy.

Sometimes you'd do anything to lull your active baby to sleep. Its kick wakes you up in the middle of the night. The continual *thump, thump, swoosh* is annoying as you try to concentrate on work. An elbow to your bladder or a swift heel to your rib cage seems anything but marvelous. Then, when your baby quiets, you worry. Is the baby okay? You poke at your belly. Hey, little one, wake up! Poke, poke. Are you sleeping, tiny baby? Dreaming? Growing? Then you feel that marvelous internal whirl of assurance, and you sigh with relief.

Occasionally you get to share the miracle with others. But when you say, "Put your hand here," the baby seems to start a game of hide-and-seek. Baby stills, hiding, as your mate, friend, or older child waits impatiently. Just when they draw their hands away—boom! Baby kicks, winning the game again.

The internal dance you share with your baby is, for the most part, yours alone. It's one of God's special gifts to mothers, a side effect of the Miracle Journey that will long outshine even the darkest of pregnancy's discomforts.

Marvel in it. Rejoice as you feel the miracle of life.

Let each movement bring you joy!

Let your child's internal playtime rejuvenate and excite you.

Let this special communion draw you closer to your baby. In moments alone, tell your child your hopes, dreams, and imaginings. Your baby already has the ability to listen.

Most of all, cherish this precious time when you hold your child so securely close to your heart.

When You Move Inside Me, It Makes Me Feel . . .

For as soon as I heard the sound of your greeting, the child in my womb leaped for joy.
—Luke 1:44

Day 1

When Elizabeth heard Mary's greeting, the child leaped in her womb. And Elizabeth was filled with the Holy Spirit and exclaimed with a loud cry, "Blessed are you among women, and blessed is the fruit of your womb." *Luke 1:41-42*

_____

_____

Day 2

Blessed is she who believed that there would be a fulfillment of what was spoken to her by the Lord. *Luke 1:45*

_____

_____

Day 3

The Mighty One has done great things for me, and holy is his name. His mercy is for those who fear him from generation to generation. *Luke 1:49-50*

_____

_____

Day 4

I have calmed and quieted my soul, like a weaned child with its mother; my soul is like the weaned child that is with me. *Psalm 131:2*

_____

_____

Day 5

Job would send and sanctify [his children], and he would rise early in the morning and offer burnt offerings according to the number of them all; for Job said, "It may be that my children have sinned, and cursed God in their hearts." This is what Job always did. *Job 1:5*

_____

Day 6

The Lord commanded our ancestors to teach his laws to their children; that the next generation might know them, the children yet unborn, and rise up and tell them to their children, so that they should set their hope in God, and not forget the works of God, but keep his commandments. *Psalm 78:5-7, adapted*

Day 7

Unless the Lord builds the house, those who build it labor in vain. Unless the Lord guards the city, the guard keeps watch in vain. *Psalm 127:1*

_____

_____

Pop quiz: Are you praying daily for your child? Are you praying for other family members who will need to adjust to a new baby? Record greetings to the unborn on a videotape.

_____

Michael's job was to plant the seed.
Then he sat back and proudly watched us grow.

$\mathcal{M}$EN—they come in all shapes, sizes, attitudes, and degrees of sensitivity. The worst thing you can do is to compare your man's actions during the Miracle Journey to those of your friend's "perfect" man.

Remember, God wired men different from women, and we've each been given distinct stereotypes by our culture. We commonly expect that:

Men think. Women feel.

Men think, "My wife finally looks pregnant."

Women feel, "I'm fat and have permanently lost my attraction and appeal."

Men think, "My pregnant wife has a problem concentrating and making choices, so I'll help her."

Women feel, "I'm losing my mind, and he's driving me crazy."

Men think, "Labor is a systematic process with an inevitable outcome."

Women feel, "I'll give you an inevitable outcome for being so practical!"

People are different. One new father may be exuberant about the expected arrival. Yet *you* may be in tears because the soon-to-be father in your family isn't obsessing two hours a day over what to name the baby. His level of enthusiasm may be several degrees lower than yours as you shop for the crib. Don't think you have the world's worst support partner or that your man will be a horrible father.

Most men make great fathers. They give their children the frolic of playtime, fearless adventure, and Daddy's special silly stuff. They lift their children high on strong shoulders for a better view of the world. They dig deeper for a better harvest, to give their offspring the start they need: good education, housing, travel, or whatever is worthwhile.

As the miracle of life takes both man and woman to conceive, so the child is blessed with father and mother. Believe it or not, *each* is teaching how to think and feel, to help make a child whole.

I planted the seed, another watered it, but God made it grow.
So neither the one who plants nor one who waters is anything,
but only God, who makes things grow.
The one who plants and the one who waters have one purpose,
and each will be rewarded according to the labor of each.
—1 Corinthians 3:6-8, NIV/NRSV, adapted

Day 1

What are human beings that you are mindful of them, mortals that you care for them? *Psalm 8:4*

_____

_____

Day 2

The Lord God said, "It is not good that the man should be alone; I will make him a helper as his partner." *Genesis 2:18*

_____

_____

Day 3

The rib that the Lord God had taken from the man he made into a woman and brought her to the man. Then the man said, "This at last is bone of my bones and flesh of my flesh; this one shall be called Woman, for out of Man this one was taken." *Genesis 2:22-23*

_____

_____

Day 4

Therefore a man leaves his father and his mother and clings to his wife, and they become one flesh. *Genesis 2:24*

_____

_____

Day 5

Taste and see that the Lord is good; happy are those who take refuge in him. O fear the Lord, you his holy ones, for those who fear him have no want. *Psalm 34:8-9*

_____

_____

Day 6

Husbands, love your wives, just as Christ loved the church and gave himself up for her. *Ephesians 5:25*

_____

_____

_____

Day 7

The older women . . . may encourage the young women to love their husbands, to love their children, to be self-controlled, chaste, good managers of the household, kind, submissive to their husbands. . . . Likewise, encourage younger men to be self-controlled. *Titus 2:3-6*

_____

_____

Pop quiz: Write a love letter to your husband and secretly tuck it into his briefcase or lunch box or under his pillow.

"Sex"—remember? . . .
It's how we got in this situation in the first place.
—Deborah Dee Grizzard

*T*HE stereotypes tell us: Men, like microwaves, just think the word *sex* and, bing, they're ready. Women, like Crock-Pots, have to s-l-o-w-l-y think about sex and heat up to it.

Here's a news flash: Sex is 99 percent mental, and sex while pregnant can trigger even more mental gymnastics. There are so many hang-ups about sex during pregnancy that we could dangle our toes in the proverbial intimacy pool until the water is ice cold before we plunge back into the enjoyable activity that got us here in the first place.

Your pre-parenthood brains are suddenly on overload. Your husband worries about the mechanics, the method, and the third set of eyes and ears between the two of you. You wonder if it will hurt, if you will hurt the baby, or if the image of your maternal body will hurt your sex appeal. All this thinking is definitely hurting your sex life.

It's time to drop the pretenses, the fear fences, the games of silent action and avoidance. Talk about it. Find a private, nonthreatening environment. Try talking through your fears with the lights off before you fall asleep one night.

Unless your doctor has told you to abstain, there is no reason why you should avoid intimacy. Cuddle, touch, and find each other again in new experiences. Regardless of your belly size, most husbands find nothing to complain about in a blossoming bustline. So concentrate on the positive new aspects of your body and tell your mate about your areas of sensitivity.

Many women joyfully admit that their bodies become more receptive and sensitive while they are pregnant, and lovemaking becomes more satisfying than ever before. Since you're no longer worrying about birth control, you might discover a freedom you've never been able to enjoy. In the later months, there is the added dimension of having to become a bit creative when it comes to positions.

So, laugh together, fumble around, stroke, pet, and reposition yourselves as you rejoice in the awesome gift the heavenly Father has given you in the intimacy of marriage.

The two will become one flesh.
—Ephesians 5:31

Day 1

Come, let us take our fill of love until morning; let us delight ourselves with love. *Proverbs 7:18*

_____

_____

_____

Day 2

Let him kiss me with the kisses of his mouth! For your love is better than wine. *Song of Solomon 1:2*

_____

_____

_____

Day 3

Then David consoled his wife Bathsheba, and went to her, and lay with her; and she bore a son, and he named him Solomon. The Lord loved him. *2 Samuel 12:24*

_____

_____

_____

Day 4

Do not forsake her, and she will keep you; love her, and she will guard you. *Proverbs 4:6*

_____

_____

_____

Day 5

So Jacob served seven years for Rachel, and they seemed to him but a few days because of the love he had for her. *Genesis 29:20*

_____

_____

_____

Day 6

Then Isaac brought her into his mother Sarah's tent. He took Rebekah, and she became his wife; and he loved her. So Isaac was comforted after his mother's death. *Genesis 24:67*

_____

_____

_____

Day 7

When a man is newly married, he shall not go out with the army or be charged with any related duty. He shall be free at home one year, to be happy with the wife whom he has married. *Deuteronomy 24:5*

_____

_____

Sixth Month

Weeks 25~28

Prayer for the Child

O Lord, this month you've covered our child's thin, red, wrinkled skin with a fine, soft hair called lanugo. Let me eat balanced, nutritious meals as you pour crucial nutrients into a tiny body that is undergoing rapid growth. Every organ system is continuing to develop as this still-tiny fetus stretches to 11-14 inches and weighs almost a pound and a half. Create a willingness in this child to never stop stretching and learning. Gift this child with the desire to know our Creator from an early age. Give our child a peaceful spirit, a tender heart, and a passion to be like Christ. Amen.

Prayer for the Mother

Creator God, I'm gaining weight by the minute. At times this makes me panic and feel guilt-ridden because of the sweet things I put in my mouth. Give me self-control to do what's right in the area of eating and exercise. Reassure me, Father, that this month is typically the time of greatest weight gain. And I do feel it! These growing-pain stitches in my side are miserable at times. Help me find ways to relax. Let me take quiet time to meditate and rejoice in this child playing and dancing within my body. These are moments to cherish. This is life! Within me is the Creator's miracle you're sharing with us. Let me draw ever closer to you and forge a relationship like none I've ever had with my precious God before. I delight in seeing your attributes anew, holy Father. Amen.

It's Time

Sign up to take a childbirth class. It's better to plan ahead than to be caught unprepared for the big event. Check with your doctor or local hospital for a schedule, and read up on the many labor and delivery techniques. You'll be surprised by the different ways of labor and delivery. Researching your options prepares you and your husband to choose the method that's right for you.

Bible Study

The woman of Proverbs 31 seems like *Mission Impossible* to most of us. Remember that the key to these verses is balance. God is not looking for perfection in us, but for the progress of a willing heart. Open your heart to the Father and see what areas of your character need refining. Praise him for the character strengths you possess, and ask him for help with your weaknesses. List some qualities in Proverbs 31 that you would like God to begin refining in you, to prepare you for motherhood.

_____

_____

_____

Her children arise and call her blessed; her husband also, and he praises her: "Many women do noble things, but you surpass them all." . . .A woman who fears the Lord is to be praised.
—Proverbs 31:28-30, NIV

69

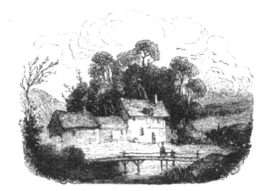

I belong to my lover, and his desire is for me.
Come, my lover, let us go to the countryside,
let us spend the night in the villages.
Let us go early to the vineyards
to see if the vines have budded,
if their blossoms have opened,
and if the pomegranates are in bloom—
there I will give you my love.
—Song of Solomon 7:10-12, NIV

*I*SN'T it time to go to your favorite place, your secret place, a quiet place, with the love of your life? Oh, yes, my friend, it is time to laugh, relax, and love. You are in the middle months of the Miracle Journey. There is no better time than the present to get away from it all. After your doctor gives you permission to travel, plan a trip. This last getaway vacation doesn't have to be a world tour or a two-week stay in the tropics. What's important is that you take the time to be alone with your husband, rejuvenating your marriage, falling deeper in love, relaxing in each other's peaceful companionship, and doing something you enjoy.

You're feeling great, and your body has yet to become a burden. In a few months, your arms, as well as your time, will be full with the baby. It may be years before you catch another opportunity to be completely alone with your spouse on a getaway.

Don't worry about showing that cute little tummy bulge on the beach. Get real! After all, you're pregnant, even if no one can tell by looking at you. When I was six months pregnant, I tried wearing a maternity swimsuit. But with just a small budding bulge, I looked ridiculously frumpy. So I went with my stylish swimwear and quickly dismissed my plumpness. I loved lying on the beach, hearing the waves, and feeling the ocean breeze. I was engulfed in my favorite author's latest high-drama suspense thriller, sipping fresh juice, and eating my fill of fresh seafood as Mike and I cast secret smiles and nipped newlywed kisses again.

We spent another long weekend in the mountains, where we often go to dream and plan and appreciate the glory of God's creation. The time there granted peace and a sense of new confidence in our future family.

Wherever you go—whether someplace new or your favorite old standby—make the time count. I hope that your last getaway vacation before motherhood arrives is your most fulfilling. Cherish the time, record it with pictures and written memories, and cleave to your husband and your God. Celebrate your blessings and look ahead to the conclusion of your Miracle Journey.

The Lord said, "My presence will go with you,
and I will give you rest."
—Exodus 33:14

Day 1

Six days you shall work, but on the seventh day you shall rest; even in plowing time and in harvest time you shall rest. *Exodus 34:21*

_____

_____

_____

Day 2

The Lord answered her . . ., "You are worried and distracted by many things; there is need of only one thing." *Luke 10:41-42*

_____

_____

_____

Day 3

Now the Lord my God has given me rest on every side; there is neither adversary nor misfortune. *1 Kings 5:4*

_____

_____

_____

Day 4

A sabbath rest still remains for the people of God; for those who enter God's rest also cease from their labors as God did from his. *Hebrews 4:9-10*

_____

_____

Day 5

Then he said to them, "Go your way, eat the fat and drink sweet wine and send portions of them to those for whom nothing is prepared, for this day is holy to our Lord; and do not be grieved, for the joy of the Lord is your strength." *Nehemiah 8:10*

_____

_____

Day 6

Thus says the Lord: Stand at the crossroads, and look, and ask for the ancient paths, where the good way lies; and walk in it, and find rest for your souls. *Jeremiah 6:16*

_____

_____

Day 7

Let the heavens be glad, and let the earth rejoice, and let them say among the nations, "The Lord is king!" *1 Chronicles 16:31*

_____

_____

ONE long-lasting and important thing you give your child is a name. Deciding on the right name can be one of the biggest challenges of your pregnancy. Eventually your name may sum you up in people's minds. By your actions and character, you fill out the meaning of your name, which others then use in perceiving who you are. You don't want to choose a name that will be a burden for your child. Some names are a good inheritance. Others have been ruined because of association with particular characters. Everyone is biased toward or against each name.

Certain names, like songs, evoke strong memories. What your mom, best friend, or even husband loves, you might hate. That's okay. What's important is that both parents are happy with the final choice. You need to make sure everyone understands that the two human creators of the baby-to-be have the sole privilege of making the final name choice!

Like my friend, you might find yourself obsessing over names. Don't get frustrated. There hasn't been a person born yet who lived without a name or label of some sort. So how do you go about selecting the right name for your child?

Start by praying. God already has a name for your little one, so listen as you begin to brainstorm. Put a piece of blank paper on your refrigerator with "girl" and "boy" written on the top line. (Unless you are completely certain of the sex, search for both.) Then list any name you hear that sounds interesting. Let friends and family join in the idea-generating process and fill the page. Search through name books. Watch the credits on television shows and movies. Take advantage of a beautiful day to walk through a cemetery—it's one of the best places in the world to find interesting names. As your roster expands, if you or your mate sees a name on the list you don't like, cross it off. Keep the brainstorming list going. During week 31, I'll list some ways to help you narrow down the choices.

If my child could be an animal, that would be

_____

If my child could be an element of nature, that would be

_____

If my child could be a color, that would be

_____

If my child could be a texture, that would be

_____

The character trait I most want to instill in my child is

_____

If my child is a boy, the most important thing about his name would be

_____

If my child is a girl, the most important thing about her name would be

_____

I found myself perplexed with finding the right name for my future child.
A boy needed a strong name, a girl—feminine, but strong.
Nothing we came up with was right … or agreeable.
In the end, my daughter came home from the hospital as "Baby girl Turk."
On her fourth day, she was Marissa.
—Bren Turk

72

The Lord called me before I was born, while I was in my mother's womb he named me.
—Isaiah 49:1

Day 1

The man named his wife Eve, because she was the mother of all living. *Genesis 3:20*

_____

_____

_____

Day 2

A good name is to be chosen rather than great riches, and favor is better than silver or gold. *Proverbs 22:1*

_____

_____

_____

Day 3

Your name is perfume poured out; therefore the maidens love you. *Song of Solomon 1:3*

_____

_____

_____

Day 4

Do not fear, for I am with you; I will bring your offspring from the east, and from the west I will gather you; . . . everyone who is called by my name, whom I created for my glory, whom I formed and made. *Isaiah 43:5, 7*

_____

_____

73

Day 5

Leah conceived again and bore a son, and said, "This time I will praise the Lord"; therefore she named him Judah; then she ceased bearing. *Genesis 29:35*

_____

_____

_____

Day 6

For you, O God, have heard my vows; you have given me the heritage of those who fear your name. *Psalm 61:5*

_____

_____

_____

Day 7

The name of the Lord is a strong tower; the righteous run into it and are safe. *Proverbs 18:10*

_____

_____

_____

Meditation~Envisioning Your Child

Find a quiet place. A favorite place. A moment in time.

Now close your eyes and cradle your belly with your hands. Caress your child, circling your hands, breathing deep and slow.

Feel the tightness of your skin, the resiliency of your belly. Imagine the warm waters of your womb.

Can you hear the heartbeat? Listen.

Now see your child. The lunar white or dusky glow of its skin, the oh-so-tiny limbs, the orbs of its eyes. Does your baby have its father's nose? Its mother's mouth? The family chin? Let your mind create a picture of its beautiful face.

Now count its fingers. Watch as its hand stretches open and then closes into a fist. Is it resting peacefully, dreaming as your heartbeat lulls it to sleep? Or is it playing, feeling the added warmth of your touch, responding to the nearness of its mother's hands? See your child as the perfect and miraculous being it is.

Tell your child about the love you feel for its father, about the dreams you envision for its life, about the hopes you have as its mother. End your time together with a special prayer.

This is what I saw:

_____

_____

_____

_____

This is what I hoped:

_____

_____

_____

_____

This is what I prayed:

_____

_____

_____

_____

Father, I thank you for the realization that we alone have not made this child, nor have natural processes alone. But you, Lord, are the great Creator who works within me, knitting together this tiny, precious life. How fearful and wonderful are your works. Yes, this I now know, very well. Amen.

Day 1

I will meditate on all your work, and muse on your mighty deeds. Your way, O God, is holy. What god is so great as our God? *Psalm 77:12-13*

_____

_____

Day 2

I rise before dawn and cry for help; I put my hope in your words. My eyes are awake before each watch of the night, that I may meditate on your promise. *Psalm 119:147-148*

_____

_____

Day 3

My soul is satisfied as with a rich feast, and my mouth praises you with joyful lips when I think of you . . . and meditate on you in the . . . night; for you have been my help, and in the shadow of your wings I sing for joy. *Psalm 63:5-7*

_____

_____

Day 4

We ponder your steadfast love, O God, in the midst of your temple. Your name, O God, like your praise, reaches to the ends of the earth. Your right hand is filled with victory. *Psalm 48:9-10*

_____

_____

Day 5

The child grew and became strong, filled with wisdom; and the favor of God was upon him. *Luke 2:40*

_____

_____

Day 6

For surely I know the plans I have for you, says the Lord, plans for your welfare and not for harm, to give you a future with hope. *Jeremiah 29:11*

_____

_____

Day 7

Satisfy us in the morning with your steadfast love, so that we may rejoice and be glad all our days. *Psalm 90:14*

_____

_____

Pop quiz: Make today a day of thanksgiving. If you're feeling bad, make a list of your blessings. Feeling better now? God is a gracious Giver!

_____

_____

75

*N*ATIVE Americans gave newborn children symbols as names. They chose names like Running Bear, Bright Star, and Forked Thunder. Their names came from occurrences at their birth or a special characteristic their proud parents hoped to bestow on them.

Likewise, you can study names and signs of Jesus: The Word, Emmanuel, Teacher, Wonderful Counselor, Lamb of God, Lion of Judah, Light of the World, Bright Morning Star, Bread of Life, Good Shepherd, Prince of Peace, King of kings, Lord of lords, True Vine, Branch, Gate, Narrow Way, Truth, Life, and the hen who protects her chicks. These images tell you what Christ does and who he is.

Your faith is also strengthened by the names and signs of God: our great Creator, Rock, Refuge, Strength, Strong Tower, Shade, Deliverer, Righteous Judge, I AM, Abba Father, and one who is as comforting as a mother. Your relationship with God is brought through the Holy Spirit, who is Helper, Advocate, Comforter, Power from on high, and Teacher. God is also the one who convicts the world of sin, gives birth from above, guides into all truth, and intercedes for us.

With forty-two bur oaks in my front yard, I watched through the seasons of my pregnancy as those grand trees changed from bare limbs, to brilliant buds, to leafy canopies, and finally to bursts of fall color. I knew those lofty ancient branches had stood through many years and would stretch and throw shade long after my time has come and gone. On October twenty-third, when a bounty of oak seeds littered the fallen leaves, I awkwardly stooped to pick up a tiny acorn. Compared to its parent, that acorn was little more than a promise. But to me, on the day my son was to be born, it was a symbol of all I hoped and dreamed a little boy would one day grow to be.

For you, maybe it's a special star that twinkles brightly each night. It might be a lofty hawk that rides the wind or a wolf that sings to heaven. It could be the unique magic of a snowflake, the promise of a rainbow, the dance of the rain, the caress of the wind, or the courage of a tender flower. Perhaps it's the fruit of the vineyard, the faith of the mustard seed, or the perseverance of the olive branch. Search your heart, look around your world, and find an emblem of significance that will be a special symbol for your child and a visual reminder of your dedication to prayer for your child.

My child's special symbol is

_____

The meaning behind it is

_____

_____

_____

_____

Even the mighty oak began as a tiny acorn that held its ground.
—Linda Davis

And he was strong as the oaks.
—Amos 2:9, KJV

Day 1

God said, "This is the sign of the covenant I am making between me and you and every living creature with you, a covenant for all generations to come: I have set my rainbow in the clouds, and it will be the sign of the covenant between me and the earth." *Genesis 9:12-13, NIV*

_____

_____

Day 2

Give me a sign of your goodness, that my enemies may see it and be put to shame, for you, O Lord, have helped me and comforted me. *Psalm 86:17, NIV*

_____

_____

Day 3

Ask a sign of the Lord your God; let it be deep as Sheol or high as heaven. *Isaiah 7:11*

_____

_____

Day 4

It is I, Jesus. . . . I am the root and the descendant of David, the bright morning star. *Revelation 22:16*

_____

_____

Day 5

More majestic than the thunders of mighty waters, more majestic than the waves of the sea, majestic on high is the Lord! *Psalm 93:4*

_____

_____

Day 6

The Lord is your keeper; the Lord is your shade at your right hand. *Psalm 121:5*

_____

_____

Day 7

For the Lord, the Most High, is awesome, a great king over all the earth. . . . He chose our heritage for us, the pride of Jacob whom he loves. *Psalm 47:2, 4*

_____

_____

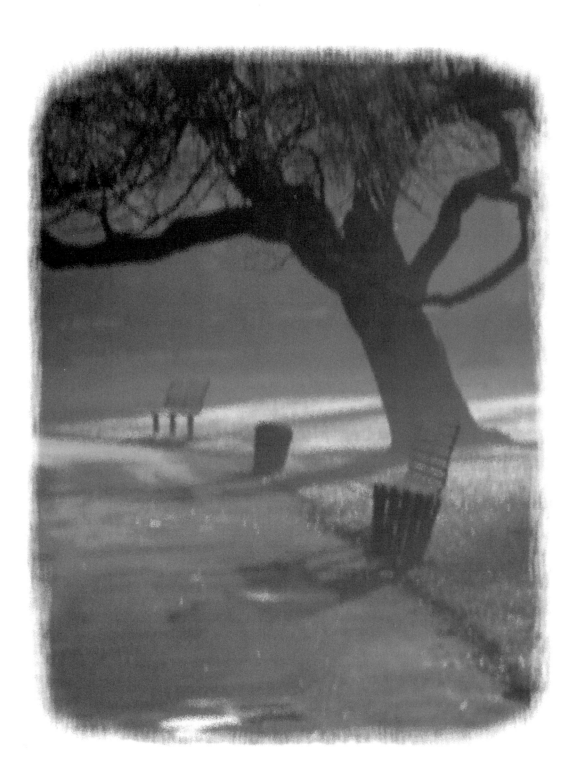

Third Trimester

Being Prepared

Are you prepared to go into unexpected labor at any time?

Complete your list of phone numbers, for making calls announcing baby's arrival (see page 112). Prepare your hospital bag and make a checklist of items you want to take, such as camera, film, pillow, music, etc. (see page 112).

Talk to your doctor and decide what steps to take if you suspect you are in labor. Plan your travel route to the hospital. Know where to go when you arrive. Have a backup coach ready in case the dad is not available to help during labor. Have child-care set up for your other children during the hospital stay.

Complete a birthing class. Research labor options. With your doctor, make your plan for delivery. Through prayer, exercise, and writing each day in your journal, prepare your mind, body, and spirit for labor and for your new life after pregnancy.

Planning and Doing

Are you preparing co-workers for your maternity leave?

Are your older children expecting the new baby? Have they taken sibling classes?

Do you have the nursery ready? Are you gathering the layette pieces?

Do you have a wish list for baby showers?

Are you researching names and keeping a running list of ideas?

Have you selected birth announcements? Have you made your address list?

Prepare some meals and freeze them to use during your recovery time.

Goal-Setting

Reconfirm the lifestyle changes you vowed in week 5.

Are you getting extra rest and saying no when necessary? Is your weight gain on target? Are you still exercising, eating healthful foods, and drinking extra water?

Are you on budget? Are you saving for the things you deem important and spending some of that savings on baby's future needs?

Keeping a Journal

Don't stop now! These last three months bring some of the most miraculous events. Record every grumble, tear, laugh, hiccup, and heartburn. Recommit yourself to writing in your journey daily as you grow and stretch spiritually. Record the milestones: The chosen names; the loss of your belly button; the innovative way you and your mate now become intimate; the first thing you buy for baby; the way you personalized the breathing exercises in childbirth class; and your questions for your next doctor's appointment. You're almost there!

Seventh Month

Weeks 29~32

Prayer for the Child

O Lord, your miracle in me is now fifteen inches long and weighs three pounds. Our baby never seems to stop kicking and stretching, pushing as if it needs more playground space. I haven't much room left, little one, but I'm so excited to feel your marvelous hiccups. Thank you, Lord, for the gift of this child's five senses. Inside my womb, your miracle can cry, hear, and open and close its eyes. Grant eyes that are curious about the beauty of your world, and ears that listen and long to learn. This little one can suck its thumb and often does so. Help us give your child security and welcome in entering this world, through our unconditional love that we have learned from you, Lord. Remind me to drink my milk. The baby needs it as the tiny bones begin to harden. Bless this child with strength and a desire to seek your righteousness. Amen.

Prayer for the Mother

Heavenly Father, I feel like every muscle and bone is straining under the incredible growth of this baby. There seems to be no space that isn't filled. My ankles, ah, they are so swollen that I should float, Lord, and my belly—well, that goes without saying. But aren't my breasts big enough now? You surely must have a sense of humor. Help me to keep mine. Lord, lead me to a moisturizer that will help my itchy tummy. I feel as if I'm full of complaints. Forgive me, holy Father. Let me remember that this is your miracle I carry. You are my sovereign God. As my apprehensions about motherhood loom ahead, let me remember that you are faithful; you will provide what I need to succeed in being the mother you have called me to be. I've learned that I did not make this child; the child is making me, through your mighty hand, to be more than I ever thought I could be. Amen.

Planning

Prepare for birth. Make a plan and a checklist. Pack your bag. Put a towel, a trash bag, and a change of clothes in the car and in your desk at work, to use in case your water breaks. Be ready for anything!

Bible Study

Read Mary's Magnificat in Luke 1:46-55. Why does Mary say she will be called blessed? Why would you say you are blessed? Write a prayer, thanking God for those blessings.

_____

_____

_____

The Mighty One
has done great
things for me,
and holy is his
name.
His mercy is for
those who fear him
from generation to
generation.
—Luke 1:49-50

As the mother of six children, I can tell you:
change is certain, laundry is constant,
all things will pass, and stretch marks will fade.
—Linda Werner

HE risk of stretch marks terrified me, so I developed a plan of attack. This is
the method in my madness: I found a moisturizer with the composition of
Crisco, then zealously greased my whole body twice a day, applying three or four coats
to belly, buttocks, and thighs. I counted the application successful by the degree to
which clothing stuck to my coated body.

I was religious about this ritual. My vanity required it. After the birth of my first
son, I walked away proudly with one small stretch mark, and my method validated.
When my second pregnancy began, I again went about like a greased pig smelling of
cocoa butter. I was sure I would come away with my flesh as unmarked as a young
girl's. Was I wrong! My second son nestled down in my right hip and refused to rise,
thus ballooning my football-shaped belly from hipbone to hipbone. My skin had no
choice but to s-t-r-e-t-c-h, and alas, I have assorted beauty marks on both hips to
remind me.

You might as well reckon with your chances: the tattoo of motherhood, better
known as stretch marks, will be given to 90 percent of all pregnant women. It doesn't
matter how expensive and miracle-moisturizing your lotion or how dedicated your ritual of application.

To help minimize stretch marks, eat a balanced diet, and do doctor-approved
exercise to insure a steady, gradual weight gain. Drink lots of water to keep the skin
hydrated, and use lotion at least once a day. To get the most penetration from your
moisturizing lotion, apply it when your skin is still damp from a bath or shower.

Most important, remember that those dark lines will eventually fade to faint silver spiderwebs that only you will notice. Turn disappointment to joy. You earned your
stretch marks! You are God's vessel, privileged with carrying a child of the great
Creator, and granted a blessed seal in the passage of the Miracle Journey.

In time, your baby girl will be a woman, your son a man. Your eyes will look at
that child in awe, unable to believe how fast he or she grew up. Then your fingers
will trace the subtle stretch marks, the tattoo of motherhood that reminds you, "Yes, I
carried this child within me. Once upon a time, I took the Miracle Journey."

Rejoice in today. Cherish the awesomeness of your blooming body, for the child
will be born, and you will again be you alone. All that will be left are a few faded
lines to remind you—and your child!

Day 1

He has taken me to the banquet hall, and his banner over me is love. *Song of Solomon 2:4, NIV*

_____

_____

_____

Day 2

Turn my eyes away from worthless things; preserve my life according to your word. *Psalm 119:37, NIV*

_____

_____

_____

Day 3

You are altogether beautiful, my love; there is no flaw in you. *Song of Solomon 4:7*

_____

_____

_____

Day 4

There is nothing better for mortals than to eat and drink, and find enjoyment in their toil. This also, I saw, is from the hand of God; for apart from him who can eat or who can have enjoyment? *Ecclesiastes 2:24-25*

_____

_____

Day 5

Charm is deceitful, and beauty is vain, but a woman who fears the Lord is to be praised. *Proverbs 31:30*

_____

_____

_____

Day 6

Tell the next generation that this is God, our God forever and ever. He will be our guide forever. *Psalm 48:13-14*

_____

_____

_____

Day 7

Jesus said to the woman, "Your faith has saved you; go in peace." *Luke 7:50, adapted*

_____

_____

_____

*B*ED *rest!* That dreaded term may be heard at any time during the Miracle Journey. For some, the first trimester is a delicate time. Less is more, and bed rest assures that you give your body the best chance to proceed. Sometimes bed rest comes as a shock. Everything seemed to be fine yesterday, and suddenly your body is sending up red flags of warning. "You're doing too much! Slow down! I can't keep up!"

Some of us become so used to being pregnant that we just keep going and adding and doing, as if we weren't otherwise occupied. I know that was my problem. I had so much on my proverbial plate that one more spoonful of traffic jam, in my hour commute, could start contractions.

One night I paced the floors, hoping to stop what we thought was false labor. Then in the morning, I wanted to deny that there ever was a problem. Feeling fine, I went into the doctor's office. I felt apologetic, embarrassed that the staff might think I was a cry-wolf type of pregnant woman. The next thing I knew, I was strapped to a monitor. A concerned doctor was talking to his nurses like a TV doctor on *ER*. "Complete bed rest," he commanded sternly. My loving compartmentalized husband wanted this clarified into two lists of what's allowed and what isn't. The doctor crossed his arms and narrowed his eyes: "She must not do anything except rest in bed."

Surely, I thought, *I can go into work and wrap things up. Listen, I have closets to clean out, drawers to organize, and casseroles to freeze. There's a baby coming, after all.* But once I talked with the pediatrician about the challenges to be endured by a baby born at thirty weeks, nothing but bed rest seemed important. My choices that day would affect my baby for all its tomorrows.

Preterm labor became my Miracle Journey obstacle to conquer, and my bridge over it was complete bed rest. I released all the things still left to be done before our baby came. I concentrated on getting through one more day to reach the goal of thirty-seven weeks. I found books to read, Christmas stockings to sew, and priceless quiet time to treasure. I had time I'd always wanted to have before but could rarely catch, time to draw close to my Lord.

At this stage, you never know what tomorrow will bring. This is why it's so important to plan. Your work associates know where things are because you've prepared them and left paper trails for them to follow. You have already planned what to do with the baby's siblings, and that program is ready to pop up on your life's computer at the trip of a finger. Your hospital bag is packed and in the car, along with a towel (in case your water breaks), phone list (of all the people to be called), and camera (for the special first moments).

Bed rest is the red light that stops life as you have known it. Being still makes you stop and slowly, delicately, and precisely place one foot in front of the other, taking one step at a time to the destination of your Miracle Journey.

"Complete bed rest," my doctor said bluntly. In other words, my life had just come to a skidding stop.
—*Anita Gustafson*

84

Be still, and know that I am God!
—*Psalm 46:10*

Day 1

"Quiet! Be still!" Then the wind stopped, and it became completely calm. *Mark 4:39, NCV*

_____

_____

_____

Day 2

Be still before the Lord, and wait patiently for him. . . . Do not fret—it leads only to evil. *Psalm 37:7-8*

_____

_____

_____

Day 3

The Lord will fight for you, and you have only to keep still. *Exodus 14:14*

_____

_____

_____

Day 4

He said, "My presence will go with you, and I will give you rest." *Exodus 33:14*

_____

_____

_____

85

Day 5

Come to me, all you that are weary and are carrying heavy burdens, and I will give you rest. *Matthew 11:28*

_____

_____

_____

Day 6

For everything there is a season, and a time for every matter under heaven. *Ecclesiastes 3:1*

_____

_____

_____

Day 7

Like a lion they crouch and lie down, like a lioness—who dares to rouse them? *Numbers 24:9, NIV*

_____

_____

_____

_____

*L*OOK at your list of names and narrow down the choices, considering many angles.

Number of names: Most forms call for first, middle, and last names, but there's no law that says names must come in threes. The most important rule is to make the combined names flow. Your surname is the fixed part of the equation, so start from there.

Sounds: Say your surname. What sounds don't flow? What sounds do?

Rhythms: Unequal numbers of syllables create pleasing rhythms. When first and last names have an equal number of syllables, a middle name with a different syllable count creates a nice balance.

Popularity: Popular names are widely accepted by others and shared by many. Research shows that most people are ready to like those who have popular names before they've met them.

Uniqueness: A distinctive and creative name will set your child apart from the crowd. However, a name that is *too* eccentric may embarrass your child. If you choose a unique name for your baby, pair it with another, more common name, an alternative to use later in life if desired.

Meaning: Most names do have meanings. If you're having trouble choosing between names, research the meanings of several names to help solidify your choice.

Namesakes: It is a compliment to the person the baby is named after. Yet remember that the child must live with that choice while growing up. Ask "Junior" friends how they feel about being namesakes.

Pronunciation: Can people pronounce the name by looking at its spelling?

Spelling: Before giving a name a creative spelling, ask yourself, "Do I want my child to have to spell out a name throughout life?" Ordinary spellings may be boring, but they have common sense behind them and are easier to handle.

Initials: What do the initials spell? Is it embarrassing or pleasant?

Stereotypes: Check for both positive and negative associations.

Nicknames: Consider nicknames that could be drawn from the chosen name. Do you like them? If you like *Michael* but hate *Mike*, be prepared to tell people that the chosen name should not be shortened.

Test it: Watch for bad rhythms, puns, and ways the name could be used in playground teasing. A person's identity is closely connected to one's name; safeguard your child from hurts. Kids can be cruel.

Wait and see: Sometimes a baby comes into the world and just doesn't look like the name you've selected. Have several names that are acceptable to both parents ready for baby's arrival.

Beware: Not all will love the "perfect" name you select. If someone turns up a nose at the name, that's okay. Your baby is not theirs to name.

Our favorite names:

Boy _____

Girl _____

What's in a name? That which we call a rose By any other word would smell as sweet; So Romeo would, were he not Romeo call'd.
—Shakespeare, in Romeo and Juliet

86

Thus says the Lord, he who created you, who formed you, . . : Do not fear, for I have redeemed you; I have called you _____. You are mine.
—Isaiah 43:1, adapted

Day 1

They made signs to his father, how he would have him called. And he asked for a writing table, and wrote, saying, His name is John. And they marveled all. *Luke 1:62-63, KJV*

Day 2

They shall put my name upon the children of Israel; and I will bless them. *Numbers 6:27, KJV*

Day 3

Jesus entered a certain village, where a woman named Martha welcomed him into her home. She had a sister named Mary, who sat at the Lord's feet and listened to what he was saying. *Luke 10:38-39, adapted*

Day 4

For as his name is, so is he. *1 Samuel 25:25*

Day 5

I will cause your name, O king, to be celebrated in all generations; therefore the peoples will praise you forever and ever. *Psalm 45:17, adapted*

Day 6

The man said, "You shall no longer be called Jacob, but Israel, for you have striven with God and with humans, and have prevailed." *Genesis 32:28*

Day 7

I will thank you forever, because of what you have done. In the presence of the faithful I will proclaim your name, for it is good. *Psalm 52:9*

Pop quiz: What has God done for you so that you can proclaim his name?

Have you not known? Have you not heard? The Lord is the everlasting God, the Creator of the ends of the earth. He does not faint or grow weary. . . . But those who wait for the Lord shall renew their strength, they shall mount up with wings like eagles, they shall run and not be weary, they shall walk and not faint. —Isaiah 40: 28, 31

TIRED? Fatigued? Weak? Are you dozing off amid the office hubbub, napping away the entire afternoon, and tumbling into bed by eight o'clock? Never in your life have you needed more strength. You are treading with a heavy belly on the increasingly steep climb of the Miracle Journey. Life doesn't hand out handicapped car stickers simply because you are pregnant. Stress doesn't stop; trials don't detour around pregnant women.

I watched a family go through the traumatic ordeal of an unknown illness with their second child. After months of searching, they finally discovered the source of this little girl's pain. It was a tumor on the spinal cord, which surgeons removed. Tori stayed in the hospital for months of recuperation and therapy as they taught her to walk again. Through it all, my friend was pregnant. How I sympathized with and prayed for this terrific mother. I knew she was facing stress, fear, and insurmountable odds each day. She had no time to be fatigued, to lose strength, to be impatient, or to be selfish. I asked, "How are you doing this?" With a faithful smile, she answered, "I'm not," and pointed heavenward.

Tracy Roberts was being renewed each day by the Lord's endless strength. He gave her victory over the adversity in her life so she could soar on eagle's wings. He allowed her to run and not get tired. Some days, he helped her to simply put one foot in front of the other and walk without fainting.

If you *wait* upon the Lord, pursue the Lord actively through studying his Word, prayer, and meditation, then he will also help you *walk* through the ordinary trials of each day of your Miracle Journey and not become weary.

God helped me soar when

_____

_____

_____

God helped me run when

_____

_____

_____

God helped me simply put one foot in front of the other when

_____

_____

_____

Lord, I praise you for you are strength and power and stamina and victory. Let my heart search for you that I may be renewed with your awesome energy. Lift me up on eagle's wings and let me soar as I await the gift of your coming miracle. Amen.

Day 1

I lie down and sleep; I wake again, for the Lord sustains me. *Psalm 3:5*

_____

_____

Day 2

He makes me lie down in green pastures; he leads me beside still waters; he restores my soul. He leads me in right paths for his name's sake. *Psalm 23:2-3*

_____

_____

Day 3

Then you will walk on your way securely and your foot will not stumble. If you sit down, you will not be afraid; when you lie down, your sleep will be sweet. *Proverbs 3:23-24*

_____

_____

Day 4

O my strength, I will watch for you; for you, O God, are my fortress. *Psalm 59:9*

_____

_____

Day 5

Seek the Lord and his strength; seek his presence continually. Remember the wonderful works he has done, his miracles, and the judgments he uttered. *Psalm 105:4-5*

_____

_____

Day 6

Offer to God a sacrifice of thanksgiving, and pay your vows to the Most High. Call on me in the day of trouble; I will deliver you, and you shall glorify me. *Psalm 50:14-15*

_____

_____

Day 7

He gives power to the faint, and strengthens the powerless. *Isaiah 40:29*

_____

_____

Eighth Month

Weeks 33~36

Prayer for the Child

O Lord, this month our child will reach five pounds and be up to eighteen inches in length. It doesn't have much room to roam anymore, and its kicks are fierce and strong. Often I can trace the shape of a knee, an elbow, a heel, or buttocks. It's all so wondrous that inside me, curled tight and snug, is a child. Forged from the fires of passion and formed by your very hand is our blessed baby. Through all my complaints and uncomfortable symptoms, keep this child safely tucked away until fully developed and ready to live apart from my body. Help the baby's brain to grow, its lungs to develop, and its soul to be prepared to accept its Savior. Thank you, Lord, for bringing us both this far. Thank you, Lord, for being ever faithful. Amen.

Prayer for the Mother

I think I've had Braxton Hicks contractions! Wow, Lord, it made me grab the vanity and take a shaky breath. I'm frightened about labor and the unknown. Help me to take one day at a time. Help me to put a filter on what I allow in my thoughts so I won't worry. Protect me and remind me to pray—often—as I become anxious. During this time of long days and longer nights, heighten my senses to your presence. Let my soul take delight in these last weeks that I alone hold this child. Prepare me for motherhood. Grant me wisdom, patience, and physical endurance. Be with me, Lord; be my strong Rock, my Tower, and my Shade. Amen.

Theme of the Month: Showers and Celebrations

In the Bible, rain represents God's blessings. Therefore, the word *shower* is a perfect demonstration of the blessings your friends wish to give to you. There is nothing like hearing your friends say, "O-o-o-h!" and "A-a-a-h!" about the tiny little things at a baby shower, especially when you are the honored mother. Even if this is not your first child, don't skip the maternal celebrations. Gather your girlfriends and enjoy the pastime of conversation and banqueting. Show off your nursery. Play goofy games. Mail out a survey and ask your friends and family to write down their best baby advice or a treasured baby memory. Have a contest to guess the baby's arrival date, and give the winner a night of baby-sitting the new arrival! Have fun! Celebrate! Involve those close to you in your miracle expectations.

Bible Study: To Finish the Race

This month, study Hebrews 12:1-3. How can you fix your eyes upon Jesus, to finish the race?

I have fought the
good fight,
I have finished
the race,
I have kept the faith.
—2 Timothy 4:7

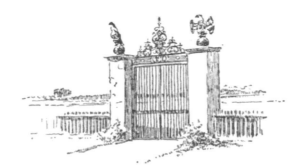

ONCE baby arrives, only the foolish take the baby out of the house without the baby bag. Any mother will tell you that the one time she darted out of the house without *The Bag* was the time disaster struck at its worst. With an infant, you can never be too prepared. Your baby bag should always be well stocked and restocked between outings.

Most mothers maintain two bags. There is the essentials bag, with diapers, wipes, and bottles. This is the small, cute, two-handled, lunch-bag shaped sack that can be grabbed at a moment's notice and holds only the most important gear. Then there is the ready-for-anything bag, which has become most modern mothers' high-fashion handbag; it holds everything but the kitchen sink.

Whichever bag you carry, the important thing is to be prepared. Know your baby. Learn her or his specific needs. Know what *must* be in The Bag. Believe me, it will only take one time at 20,000 feet in a crowded 727 to teach a new mother to always have an extra pacifier in her bag—especially if that's "the thing" that keeps her baby happy.

The Bag can be anything. You don't have to tote around a whimsical-patterned baby bag-classic done in duck motif. Nondescript totes and backpacks make great baby bags, and Dad feels a lot more comfortable toting them. (My favorite is found in the *Land's End Catalog*.)

What goes in The Bag? Anything that makes your life as a parent easier, such as the following:

Diaper essentials: Diapers, wipes, foldable pad for changing baby, plastic throw-away bags to store soiled diapers and clothing.

Mini medicine chest: diaper rash ointment, baby powder, Vaseline, infant pain reliever, drops for gas (ask your doctor), Band-Aids, antiseptic, fingernail clippers, comb, Q-Tips (travel-size items are best).

Baby garb: Complete change of clothes, receiving blanket, extra blouse for you (especially if your baby often spits up).

Baby food: Bib, burp cloth, bottles of formula unless you are breast-feeding, bottles of juice and water, pacifier. As baby grows, goodies will help keep your baby happy for longer times away from home. Ask your pediatrician for ideas.

Entertainers: Rattles, teethers, and eye-catchers galore. The trick is to find small, assorted dazzlers that you can hand out at a moment's notice. Plastic connectable rings are wonderful to chain together. Attach one end to stroller or car seat and the other to a toy. This makes keeping and retrieving toys easy. Small toys that make music at the touch of a button are lifesavers in a traffic jam. Check all of these things for safety. Discard anything that could fit into the baby's mouth or anything with small parts that could come off.

Never, I repeat, never leave the house without an extra knappie, lass. It's better to leave the house without the bairn than to be somewhere with a stink and have no means to remove it.
—*A Scottish Nanny*

92

Be shepherds of God's flock that is under your care, serving as overseers— not because you must, but because you are willing, as God wants you to be . . . eager to serve; not lording it over those entrusted to you, but being examples to the flock. And when the Chief Shepherd appears, you will receive the crown of glory that will never fade away.
—*1 Peter 5:2-4, NIV*

Day 1

Honest balances and scales are the Lord's; all the weights in the bag are his work. *Proverbs 16:11*

_____

_____

_____

Day 2

The horse is made ready for the day of battle, but the victory belongs to the Lord. *Proverbs 21:31*

_____

_____

_____

Day 3

Beware, keep alert; for you do not know when the time will come. *Mark 13:33*
Is your bag packed for the hospital? Is it in the car? Are you ready?

_____

_____

_____

Day 4

Be ready in the morning, and come up in the morning to Mount Sinai and present yourself there to me, on the top of the mountain. *Exodus 34:2*

_____

_____

_____

Day 5

Be dressed ready for action and have your lamps lit; be like those who are waiting for their master to return from the wedding banquet, so that they may open the door for him as soon as he comes and knocks. *Luke 12:35-36*

_____

_____

Day 6

In all toil there is profit, but mere talk leads only to poverty. *Proverbs 14:23*

_____

_____

_____

Day 7

It will be good for those servants whose master finds them ready, even if he comes in the second or third watch of the night. *Luke 12:38, NIV*

_____

_____

_____

93

Two are better than one,
because they have a good reward for their toil.
For if they fall, one will lift up the other;
but woe to one who is alone and falls and does not have another to help.
Again, if two lie together, they keep warm; but how can one keep warm alone?
And though one might prevail against another, two will withstand one.
A threefold cord is not quickly broken.
—Ecclesiastes 4:9-12

WHEN I learned that I was pregnant with my second child, the news was bittersweet. I had been an only child, and I longed for the gift of siblings for my firstborn. Yet, somehow, I felt I'd made some horrible mistake; I couldn't possibly love another child like I loved my precious firstborn son. How would we make certain he knew that he was just as important to us as he'd always been? How could I accept the fact that he would never again be the chief star of his parents' universe? Our most important parental love? I was frightened that somehow the new baby would hurt my son. I honestly couldn't imagine the three of us making room for a fourth in our tight family circle.

It is true that when a sibling is born, a family changes. As your family grows, a new and unique dimension is added with each child. Miraculously, the hearts of the parents and their children enlarge. We love the precious second child as fiercely as we loved our precious first. The oldest loses a part of our total attention. In return that firstborn is given the wonderful gift of love, friendship, and fulfillment only a brother or sister can bring.

Understand that the birth of a sibling is a huge change for your child. Don't make the new baby a *surprise!* Make sure to properly prepare older siblings by making them a part of the Miracle Journey as early as possible. Talk about the new baby, and help your children to understand that they are expecting a new brother or sister. You'll be surprised how receptive they can be. Our eighteen-month-old Colton surprised us all with his understanding. We told him daily that he was going to be a big brother. We'd pat my belly and tell him that's where Colton's baby was growing. When he saw his active sibling on my 16-week sonogram, he proudly declared to the entire room that the figure on the tiny screen was "Colton's baby."

We prayed each night for Colton's baby. We thanked God for his gift of a sibling and special lifelong friend. We asked the Father to help Colton accept the new baby with love and to remember that Mom and Dad would always love Colton.

Our prayers were answered. From the first instant Colton met Clay, there was never a moment of hesitancy or envy. Their love was so strong the bond of brotherhood was sowed with childlike prayers and reaped when Colton gave a precious kiss to our newborn, Clay.

Children born to a young man are like sharp arrows to defend him. Happy is the man who has his quiver full of them.
—Psalm 127:4-5, TLB

Day 1

A man of many companions may come to ruin, but there is a friend who sticks closer than a brother. *Proverbs 18:24, NIV*

_____

_____

_____

Day 2

As iron sharpens iron, so one man sharpens another. *Proverbs 27:17, NIV*

_____

_____

_____

Day 3

Each one helps the other, saying to one another, "Take courage!" *Isaiah 41:6*

_____

_____

_____

Day 4

Say to wisdom, "You are my sister," and call insight your intimate friend. *Proverbs 7:4*

_____

_____

_____

95

Day 5

For whoever does the will of my Father in heaven is my brother and sister and mother. *Matthew 12:50*

_____

_____

_____

Day 6

It is good not to . . . do anything that makes your brother or sister stumble. *Romans 14:21*

_____

_____

_____

Day 7

The faithful and beloved brother . . . is one of you. *Colossians 4:9*

_____

_____

_____

_____

May our sons in their youth be like plants full grown,
our daughters like corner pillars, cut for the building of a palace.
—Psalm 144:12

"*IS it a boy or a girl?*" How many times have you been asked? Well, answer the following questions, then tally up your score to see if the old wives' tales can really predict the color of the nursery.

You are expecting a BOY if—	*You are expecting a GIRL if—*
your hair is lustrous and bouncy.	your hair is dull and stringy.
your fanny has remained the same shape.	your fanny is enlarging.
your face has remained the same shape.	your face is fuller.
your feet get cold.	your feet are the same as before pregnancy.
you experience shortness of breath.	you're breathing easy.
your baby's heart rate is below 139 beats per minute.	your baby's heart rate is above 140 beats per minute.
you prefer to sleep on your right side.	you prefer to sleep on your left side.
you are seldom nauseated.	you are suffering from morning sickness.
you are glowing.	you are having a troublesome pregnancy.
you are craving sour and salty foods.	you are craving sweets.
you carry the baby high.	you carry the baby low.
your belly is shaped like a basketball.	your belly is shaped like a football.
you are getting kicks to the ribs.	you are getting kicks to the pelvis.

Here's an amusing test: Remove your wedding ring and tie it to a twelve-inch thread. Lie down on your back and have a friend hold the thread so the ring is a few inches above your belly. If your ring swings from hip to hip, it's a boy. If it swings from chin to toe, it's a girl.

Based on these old wives' tales, I'm having a—

BOY.   **GIRL.**

Day 1

Your wife will be like a fruitful vine within your house; your children will be like olive shoots around your table. *Psalm 128:3*

_____

_____

_____

Day 2

Come, O children, listen to me; I will teach you the fear of the Lord. *Psalm 34:11*

_____

_____

_____

Day 3

May the Lord make you increase, both you and your children. *Psalm 115:14, NIV*

_____

_____

_____

Day 4

See, everyone who uses proverbs will use this proverb about you, "Like mother, like daughter." *Ezekiel 16:44*

_____

_____

_____

Day 5

When Adam had lived one hundred thirty years, he became the father of a son in his likeness, according to his image, and named him Seth. *Genesis 5:3*

_____

_____

_____

Day 6

I will tell of the decree of the Lord: He said to me, "You are my son; today I have begotten you." *Psalm 2:7*

_____

_____

_____

Day 7

I will pour out my Spirit on your offspring, and my blessing on your descendants. They will spring up like grass in a meadow, like poplar trees by flowing streams. *Isaiah 44:3-4, NIV*

_____

_____

The righteous flourish like the palm tree,
and grow like a cedar in Lebanon.
They are planted in the house of the Lord;
they flourish in the courts of our God.
In old age they still produce fruit;
they are always green and full of sap.
—Psalm 92:12-14

Paste a
full-length
photograph
of yourself
here
at week 36.
You're almost
there!

You Are Beautiful!
So you think a woman at full term can't be beautiful?

Even if you aren't convinced, have your mate snap a photo of your bountiful maternal body
and place it here to remind you of the days you walked the Miracle Journey.
In a few months you'll be glad you captured your bountiful, beautiful, baby-full belly.

Day 1

You are altogether beautiful, my love; there is no flaw in you. *Song of Solomon 4:7*

_____

_____

_____

Day 2

You are worthy, our Lord and God, to receive glory and honor and power, for you created all things, and by your will they existed and were created. *Revelation 4:11*

_____

_____

_____

Day 3

I trust in you, O Lord; I say, "You are my God." My times are in your hand. *Psalm 31:14-15*

_____

_____

_____

Day 4

Who is this that appears like the dawn, fair as the moon, bright as the sun, majestic as the stars in procession? *Song of Solomon 6:10, NIV*

_____

_____

_____

Day 5

You are precious in my sight, and honored, and I love you. *Isaiah 43:4*

_____

_____

_____

Day 6

For where your treasure is, there your heart will be also. *Luke 12:34*

_____

_____

_____

Day 7

He has made everything beautiful in its time. *Ecclesiastes 3:11, NIV*

_____

_____

_____

Ninth Month

Weeks 37~40

Prayer for the Child

Your miracle, Lord, is gaining about a half pound a week, weighs from six to nine pounds, and is about twenty inches long. I can hardly believe all of this is tucked inside my blossomed belly. I can't imagine myself growing any bigger. The fetus usually settles head down into the birthing position, with knees against its nose and its thighs tight against its torso. Lord, help position this child correctly for a safe birth. Mature this precious one's lungs for delivery, to breathe freely once they arrive in the world. Protect this child from the dangers of delivery. Give me faith for these last weeks that I might stand on the promises I know are true. You are sovereign. You are faithful. You are with me, always. Amen.

Prayer for the Mother

Lord, I'm having a hard time getting a good night's sleep. It used to be that heartburn and inability to get a good deep breath kept me from falling asleep. Now that the baby has dropped, my bladder calls constantly, and I'm up and down all night. Are you preparing me for those early-morning feedings? Are the contractions I'm having like the *real* ones? Oh, Lord, I don't know if I'm ready for this. I'm anxious about the looming black hole of labor and delivery. Build a hedge of protection around my family and me. Let nothing prevent me from arriving safely at the hospital when my time comes. Surround me with nurses who encourage me like your angels. Grant my doctors wisdom and skill to guide your child and me through the birthing process. Fill my family and friends with the joy of sharing in your miracle. Bless my husband with peace, patience, and tolerance. Bless me with courage, endurance, and faith. Please let me never forget that you are always with me, holding my hand, prepared for anything. Let the birth of this baby glorify you in every way. Amen.

Theme of the Month: Waiting

The *waiting* is the hardest part, and calendar watching only makes it worse. Due dates will come and go for 50 percent of you. Ten percent will still be waiting two weeks after the due date. But never fear; you won't be pregnant forever. The success in waiting is to stay busy. Work on addressing birth announcement envelopes. Cook and freeze a few meals. Plan outings with friends. See the hot movie, and eat at your favorite restaurant. Seize the day and make the most of it. When you are worried and anxious, *pray*; keep a continuous conversation of prayer going all day long.

Bible Study: In the Fullness of Time

This month, study Ecclesiastes 3:1-15. God is in control of time. He cares about you and loves you. God knows when the fullness of time has come. Can you release your waiting to him?

When the fullness
of time had come,
God sent his Son,
born of a woman,
born under the law,
in order to redeem
those who were
under the law,
so that we might
receive adoption as
children.
And because you
are children, God
has sent the Spirit
of his Son
into our hearts,
crying, "Abba!
Father!"
—Galatians 4:4-6

You're home. Alone. The newborn cries.
You awkwardly pick him up. He wails.
You try feeding, burping, changing, and rocking. He cries louder.
You beg those "maternal instincts" to kick in. Nothing.
Panic builds as you pace and jiggle.
His face gets redder and redder as his cry gets louder and louder.
You try harder and harder.
Finally, you look up and sob . . .
Where is the instruction book?
—Jo Ann Dickinson

THEY handed me the baby and said, "Good luck, Mrs. Kelly!" and then wheeled me out of the hospital. I looked into the face of my sleeping son and panicked. I couldn't leave the hospital yet! What if he decided to do something besides eat or sleep? I still couldn't say the word *bath* without having a panic attack. And what if he cried? What if I couldn't stop his crying? Where *was* the instruction book? And where was his off button so I could read the instructions?

I'd gathered a library of childcare books from Dr. Spock to Dr. Dobson, but no book taught the instincts a mother must use to identify trouble and quickly respond to any situation. I felt overwhelmed by the task ahead of me; I realized I needed my maternal instincts fired up. I prayed for strong second-sense natural instincts. I prayed for wisdom, for the ability to discern and learn so I could discipline and teach my child. I, Jessica Kelly—and no other—was Colton's mother. Colton's father and I would nurture him and help form his character. We would raise this tiny boy into a man, as another link in the passage of our family. What a responsibility it suddenly was!

We have all come before these children and walked the road ahead of them. We realize that this world is not purely a place of peace and light, that it does not always vibrate with the name of the heavenly Father, with the love he intends for all of us. For this reason, the birth of children increases in us the intention and commitment to light the world with love for their sakes, to better ourselves so we can set worthy examples for them to follow. Thus we can prepare them for the days ahead when they too shall be an example for a child.

Therefore, if you are feeling a bit terrified by the awesome responsibility of parenthood, don't worry about tomorrow. Instead, pray for today. Ask for wisdom for today, and God will graciously give it. God miraculously supplies all our daily needs and prepares us for tomorrow's needs.

Lord, renew our hearts today, and purify our intentions and purposes. Teach us your ways, and show us your paths. Grant us wisdom and discernment so that we might lead our children in love. Amen.

If any of you is lacking in wisdom, ask God, who gives to all generously and ungrudgingly, and it will be given you.
—James 1:5

102

Day 1

Give me wisdom and knowledge, that I may lead this people, for who is able to govern this great people of yours? *2 Chronicles 1:10, NIV*

_____

_____

_____

Day 2

Call to me and I will answer you and tell you great and unsearchable things you do not know. *Jeremiah 33:3, NIV*

_____

_____

_____

Day 3

Where then does wisdom come from? And where is the place of understanding? . . . God understands the way to it, and he knows its place. *Job 28:20, 23*

_____

_____

_____

Day 4

So do not worry about tomorrow, for tomorrow will bring worries of its own. Today's trouble is enough for today. *Matthew 6:34*

_____

_____

Day 5

Cast your cares on the Lord and he will sustain you; he will never let the righteous fall. *Psalm 55:22, NIV*

_____

_____

Day 6

The fear of the Lord is the beginning of wisdom; all those who practice it have a good understanding. His praise endures forever. *Psalm 111:10*

_____

_____

Day 7

If you seek it like silver, and search for it as for hidden treasures—then you will understand the fear of the Lord and find the knowledge of God. For the Lord gives wisdom; from his mouth come knowledge and understanding. *Proverbs 2:4-6*

_____

_____

Everywhere I went, I was hearing headline stories:
Woman in labor 72 hours forfeits the fight to C-section.
Woman gives birth to 13 pounder—naturally.
Women gives birth on secretary's desk while whole office watches!
Labor loomed like a black hole ahead of me.
Mysterious, scary, and something I wanted to avoid at all costs!
I suddenly didn't care if this baby stayed inside me forever—
I was not giving birth!
—Lisa Stickney

AS women, we hear and tell labor stories like children swapping trading cards. It seems the bigger you grow, the bigger the legend of labor becomes. Every labor story is more horrific than the previous one. Pain is sensationalized. You visualize the impossible physics of pumpkins fitting through peashooters. After you see the show-all labor film in childbirth class, you're downright terrified.

Why does every mother feel the need to share her personal experience? Why does she tell all the gory details? Why is it chronicled again and again for whoever will listen? Come on! Physically it's the same basic process for all of us. No child has come into the world through any means other than birth. Ever since Eve, zillions of women have been doing it. So why all the stories? Why the sensationalism? And why do we all listen?

Childbirth is painful. It's grisly. It's definitely unattractive. Up until the past century, it was quite life-threatening. Labor seems like something we would want to forget, not chronicle.

Before giving birth, we can't imagine ourselves as the woman on the delivery table in the birthing video. We know there are doctors, nurses, and fathers to coach us. There are focal points, breathing techniques, and blessed epidurals to get us through the pain. We understand that we will weep and cry out that we can't do it. But we can . . . and we do!

We overcome pain by accepting it. We persevere because we realize there is no other way but forward. We try it—the hard way, the old way, the natural way— because we want to experience every sensation of giving birth. And no matter the method, painful or painfree, there is no greater means to the end. We are all decorated heroes with unique battle stories to be shared. Why? Because overcoming it all and giving life to a new person is such a great moment in your life. It is your legacy, your Miracle Journey, and it is worthy to be told and retold.

Find a Bible verse, hymn, or song lyric that you can use during labor. Type it out or memorize it. Meditate on the words to give you courage and strength.

My meditation verse:

_____

_____

The Ticopia of the Solomon Islands announce the birth of a child by saying, "A mother has given birth!" rather than "A child is born!" The Miracle Journey is your accomplishment. You have given birth!

Day 1

When a woman is in labor, she has pain, because her hour has come. But when her child is born, she no longer remembers the anguish because of the joy of having brought a human being into the world. *John 16:21*

_____

_____

Day 2

He saw that a resting place was good, and that the land was pleasant; so he bowed his shoulder to the burden, and became a slave at forced labor. *Genesis 49:15*

_____

_____

Day 3

Do you count the months till they bear? Do you know the time they give birth? They crouch down and bring forth their young; their labor pains are ended. *Job 39:2-3, NIV*

_____

_____

Day 4

Do not fear, for I am with you, do not be afraid, for I am your God; I will strengthen you, I will help you, I will uphold you with my victorious right hand. *Isaiah 41:10*

_____

_____

Day 5

For in hope we were saved. Now hope that is seen is not hope. For who hopes for what is seen? But if we hope for what we do not see, we wait for it with patience. Likewise the Spirit helps us in our weakness; for we do not know how to pray as we ought, but that very Spirit intercedes with sighs too deep for words. *Romans 8:24-26*

_____

_____

Day 6

Ask now, and see, can a man bear a child? Why then do I see every man with his hands on his loins like a woman in labor? Why is every face turned pale? Alas! that day is so great that there is none like it. It is a time of distress; yet you shall be rescued from it. Have no fear, and do not be dismayed. For I am with you, says the Lord, to save you. *Jeremiah 30:6-11, abridged, adapted*

_____

_____

Day 7

For a long time I have held my peace, I have kept still and restrained myself; now I will cry out like a woman in labor, I will gasp and pant. *Isaiah 42:14*

_____

_____

When I had my children, things were different.
Dads weren't in the delivery room and the newborn was quickly swept away.
Twelve hours later, they told me they'd be bringing the baby in.
We stood waiting at the door like kids on Christmas morning.
I was prepared for my son to look ugly, like most newborns I'd seen.
But when they presented him to me, I was immediately
overwhelmed at how beautiful he was. . . . When I held him for the first time,
I suddenly understood more about my mother than I ever had before.
Everything she had said, done, sacrificed for me—it suddenly made sense.
From the moment I held my son, I understood the boundlessness of a mother's love.
—Freyja Carlstedt

DURING the Miracle Journey, you and your husband love a surreal, faceless stranger. But once that newborn babe is placed in your arms, the darling instantaneously becomes your child. You are the mother and father. In the first moments after you give birth, many of you will actually form a stronger bond with your own parents than with your baby. The outpouring of love can seem almost overwhelming. For the first time in your lives, you truly get a glimpse of how much your parents love you. You suddenly understand their fears, burden of responsibility, and sacrifice.

As parents, you are given first-line, twenty-four-hour responsibility for the care of another person. You will impose your values, pass on your genetic strengths and weaknesses, and taint this wholly innocent child with your parental mistakes. The sheer magnitude of parenthood feels overwhelming. You quickly realize that there is no *really* perfect way of parenting. The hospital will not give you a how-to guidebook with guaranteed right answers. There are conflicting opinions about how to be good parents. What was done when you were children is now done sooner or later or not at all. You doubt and question. Your self-confidence is tested every day. But honestly, does it really matter if you bathe the baby as perfectly as the nurse did? *No!* What matters is that you nurture and develop this child with increasing confidence in your ability to guide it because you are the parents. Because you are the parents, you love this child more than anyone else on earth. Because of that love, you will know what is best for your child.

God gave this child to you. The writer of Hebrews tells us that we discipline our children for a short time as seems best to us, but God disciplines us throughout life for our good, so that we may share his holiness (Hebrews 12:10). God is therefore bigger than any of our worst parenting mistakes. If we love him, God will work all things for our children's good. God's perfect parental love is all we need. His love is our greatest gift. His love will last a lifetime.

All that I am or hope to be I owe to my angel mother.
—Abraham Lincoln

Let her love always make you happy, let her love always hold you captive.
—Proverbs 5:19, NCV

Day 1

Many waters cannot quench love, neither can floods drown it. If one offered for love all the wealth of his house, it would be utterly scorned. *Song of Solomon 8:7*

_____

_____

Day 2

Train children in the right way, and when old, they will not stray. *Proverbs 22:6*

_____

_____

Day 3

Encourage the younger women to love their husbands, to love their children, to be self-controlled, chaste, good managers of the household, kind, being submissive to their husbands, so that the word of God may not be discredited. *Titus 2:4-5*

_____

Day 4

From infancy you have known the holy Scriptures, which are able to make you wise for salvation through faith in Christ Jesus. *2 Timothy 3:15, NIV*

_____

_____

Day 5

Teach God's words to your children, talking about them when you are at home and when you are away, when you lie down and when you rise. *Deuteronomy 11:19, adapted*

_____

_____

Day 6

Sons and daughters, come and listen and let me teach you the importance of trusting the Lord. *Psalm 34:11, adapted*

_____

_____

Day 7

In the fear of the Lord one has strong confidence, and one's children will have a refuge. *Proverbs 14:26*

_____

_____

_____

I have prayed for your future since before you were born.
I leave, confident in your salvation, knowing that God has heard my prayers
and will answer them and provide for you.
I shall meet you in that perfect place where grace brings us,
and there we shall be together again, forever, with him.
—Sharon Lee

MY mother spoke these words to me days before she died of cancer. I was only sixteen and far from understanding the scope of life, death, God, or the overwhelming love parents have for their children. But during my first sixteen years, my mother was ever busy, planting, sowing, and tending the tender seeds that would grow to be her eternal gift to me.

Until I had children of my own, I did not recognize the gracious legacy my mother left within me. She mothered with love and wisdom. She taught me about the Lord, modeled the Christian life, and nurtured my early spiritual growth. She gave me roots that held through the storms of life. My mother's prayers were answered long after she passed away. Fulfilled in me, her only child, those prayers now bear fruit that is being planted in her grandchildren.

As parents, we must realize that our children are gifts, loaned to us temporarily to draw us closer to God. Our souls understand that being parents is a privilege. Therefore, we must rise to the occasion and seize the responsibility to teach these children to know, love, and serve God through their own personal relationships. We are responsible for the task of laying a foundation for spiritual growth, and we will be held accountable to God for the building we do.

We've often heard of roots and wings, of family trees and legacies. But when your life is over and you draw that last breath, what will be left a minute after you pass on? What will make it through the Father's refining fire? What jewels of reward will be in your heavenly crown?

What legacy can your husband and you leave your children?

- You can teach them about the Father.
- You can pray for them without ceasing.
- You can live a godly life that serves as a model for them to follow.

We must hold ourselves accountable to God for the gifts he has given us in the lives of our children.

I will pour out my Spirit into your children,
and my blessing on your descendants.
—Isaiah 44:3, NCV

Day 1

I have chosen him, that he may charge his children and his household after him to keep the way of the Lord by doing righteousness and justice. *Genesis 18:19*

_____

_____

Day 2

Now if you are unwilling to serve the Lord, choose this day whom you will serve. . . but as for me and my household, we will serve the Lord. *Joshua 24:15*

_____

_____

Day 3

The lines are fallen unto me in pleasant places; yea, I have a goodly heritage. *Psalm 16:6, KJV*

_____

_____

Day 4

Your children will be like jewels that a bride wears proudly. *Isaiah 49:18, NCV*

109

_____

_____

Day 5

Our children will live in your presence, and their children will remain with you. *Psalm 102:28, NCV*

_____

_____

Day 6

I will be careful to lead a blameless life. . . . I will walk in my house with a blameless heart. *Psalm 101:2, NIV*

_____

_____

Day 7

Upon you I have leaned from my birth; it was you who took me from my mother's womb. My praise is continually of you. *Psalm 71:6*

_____

_____

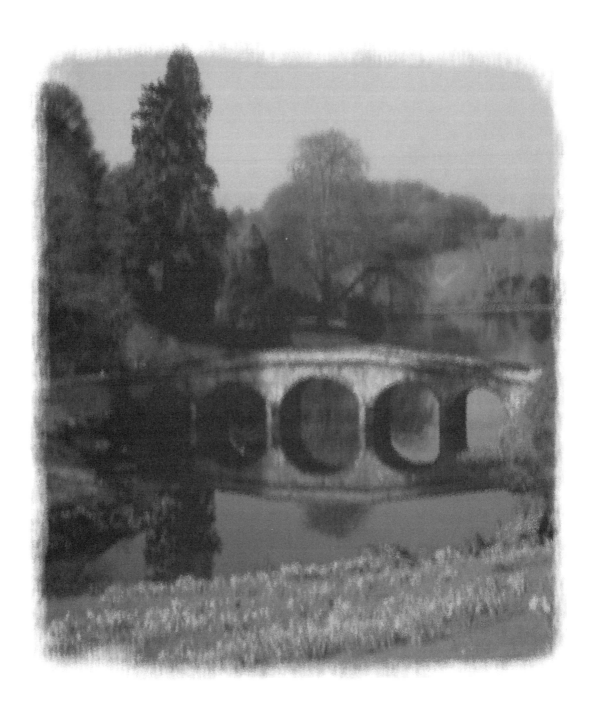

My Record of Faith

What God Taught Me During My Miracle Journey

Week 5 _____

Week 6 _____

Week 7 _____

Week 8 _____

Week 9 _____

Week 10 _____

Week 11 _____

Week 12 _____

Week 13 _____

Week 14 _____

Week 15 _____

Week 16 _____

Week 17 _____

Week 18 _____

Week 19 _____

Week 20 _____

Week 21 _____

Week 22 _____

Week 23 _____

Week 24 _____

Week 25 _____

Week 26 _____

Week 27 _____

Week 28 _____

Week 29 _____

Week 30 _____

Week 31 _____

Week 32 _____

Week 33 _____

Week 34 _____

Week 35 _____

Week 36 _____

Week 37 _____

Week 38 _____

Week 39 _____

Week 40 _____

Phone List and Hospital Preparation

Doctor _____   Number _____
                                     Number _____
Labor coach _____   Number _____
                                     Number _____
Alt. labor coach _____   Number _____
                                     Number _____
Hospital _____   Number _____
  Address _____
Childcare provider _____   Number _____
Car or cab _____   Number _____
Insurance company _____   Number _____
  Policy type _____   Number _____

Family

_____   Number _____
_____   Number _____
_____   Number _____
_____   Number _____
_____   Number _____
_____   Number _____

Friends

_____   Number _____
_____   Number _____
_____   Number _____
_____   Number _____
_____   Number _____
_____   Number _____

Other important numbers:

_____   Number _____
_____   Number _____
_____   Number _____
_____   Number _____

Checklist of items to take along to the hospital:

_____   _____
_____   _____
_____   _____
_____   _____
_____   _____
_____   _____

A Blessing for Our Child

Dear _____:

You have been such a great blessing to me because

_____

_____

_____

_____

_____

_____

If you remember only one thing that I will teach you, remember that

_____

_____

_____

_____

_____

_____

I want to always encourage you to

_____

_____

_____

_____

_____

_____

When you think of me, I hope you will remember

_____

_____

_____

_____

_____

My blessing for your life is

_____

_____

_____

_____

_____

113

*The Lord bless you
and keep you;
the Lord make his
face to shine upon
you, and be
gracious to you;
the Lord lift up his
countenance upon
you, and give you
peace.
—Numbers 6:24-26*

Thus Says the Lord

Because . . .

All scripture is inspired by God and is useful
for teaching, for reproof, for correction, and for training in righteousness,
so that everyone who belongs to God may be proficient,
equipped for every good work.
—2 Timothy 3:16-17

I felt it was essential to strengthen you daily with the Word of the living God as you prepared for motherhood. My hope is that the Spirit worked within me as I wrote this book, making my words a personal encouragement each step along the way. Peace to each of you, and congratulations on your miracle!

During the days ahead, remember,

Thus says the Lord,
who made you, who formed you in the womb and will help you:
Do not fear, . . . my servant, . . . whom I have chosen.
For I will pour water on the thirsty land, and streams on the dry ground;
I will pour my spirit upon your descendants, and my blessing on your offspring.
They shall spring up like a green tamarisk, like willows by flowing streams.
This one will say, "I am the Lord's," another will be called by the name of Jacob,
yet another will write on the hand, "The Lord's," and adopt the name of Israel.
Thus says the Lord, the King of Israel, and his Redeemer, the Lord of hosts:
I am the first and I am the last; besides me there is no god.
—Isaiah 44:2-6

Appendixes

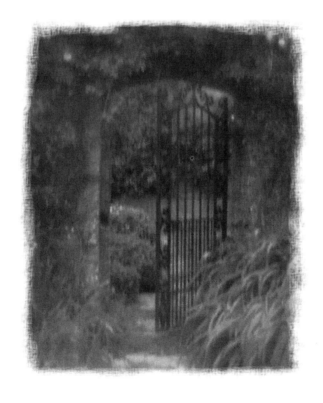

Diet

Variety is the spice of life, so here is
a variety of samplings from each of the food groups.

Protein ~ 4 daily

3 glasses of milk, 8-oz. each
31/2 oz. tuna
21/2 oz. chicken/turkey
31/2 oz. fish/shrimp
3 oz. beef, lamb, pork
3/4 cup cottage cheese
13/4 cup low-fat yogurt
5 oz. tofu (bean curd)
2 large eggs

Iron-Rich Foods ~ 1 a day

Beef
Cooked oysters
Sardines
Pumpkin seeds
Spinach
Blackstrap molasses
Dried fruit (raisins, apricots, peaches)
Legumes (peas, lentils, kidney/lima beans)

Whole Grains ~ 4 daily

1 slice whole wheat, rye, or soy bread
Brown or wild rice 1/2 cup
    oatmeal or whole-grain cereal
1/2 whole wheat bagel/English muffin
1 tortilla

Calcium ~ 4 daily

8 oz. glass of low-fat milk
2 oz. cheese
13/4 cups cottage cheese
1 cup low-fat yogurt
3/4 cup almonds

Vitamin C ~ 2 daily

1/2 grapefruit or 1/2 cup juice
1 orange or 1/2 cup juice
1/4 cantaloupe
1/2 cup strawberries
3 cups raw spinach
1/2 cup fresh broccoli
1/2 small red/green bell pepper

Fruits & Vegetables ~ 4 daily

Green Leafy, Yellow Vegetables, & Yellow Fruits
At least 1 green, 1 yellow, 1 raw

Fruits
1/8 cantaloupe
1 large peach
1/4 large mango
2 medium nectarines
2 medium apricots

Vegetables
3/4 cup broccoli
1/2 small carrot
11/2 cups Boston/romaine lettuce
1/2 cup spinach
1 large tomato
2 oz. winter squash
1/4 small yam

Diet Drill

For the next three days, write down everything you eat. On the fourth day, take your list and transpose what you ate into the food groups listed. Then evaluate how balanced your diet was and where you need to cut back or add for improvement. If you are not eating a healthful diet, have your doctor recommend a nutrition book to help you develop good eating habits. Use the quiz again to check your diet's progress.

DAY ONE

Protein	_____	(4 daily servings)
Calcium	_____	(4 daily servings)
Fruits	_____	(2-4 daily servings)
Vegetables	_____	(2-4 daily servings)
Vitamin C foods	_____	(2 daily servings)
*GL, YV, YF	_____	(3 daily servings)
Whole grains,		
Complex carbohydrates	_____	(4 daily servings)
Iron-rich foods	_____	(1 daily servings)
High-fat foods	_____	(2 daily servings)
Water	_____	(10 servings, 8-oz. each)

* Green Leafy Vegetables, Yellow Vegetables, Yellow Fruits

DAY TWO

Protein	_____	(4 daily servings)
Calcium	_____	(4 daily servings)
Fruits	_____	(2-4 daily servings)
Vegetables	_____	(2-4 daily servings)
Vitamin C foods	_____	(2 daily servings)
*GL, YV, YF	_____	(3 daily servings)
Whole grains,		
Complex carbohydrates	_____	(4 daily servings)
Iron-rich foods	_____	(1 daily servings)
High-fat foods	_____	(2 daily servings)
Water	_____	(10 servings, 8-oz. each)

DAY THREE

Proteins	_____	(4 daily servings)
Calcium	_____	(4 daily servings)
Fruits	_____	(2-4 daily servings)
Vegetables	_____	(3 daily servings)
Vitamin C foods	_____	(2 daily servings)
*GL, YV, YF	_____	(3 daily servings)
Whole grains,		
Complex carbohydrates	_____	(4 daily servings)
Iron-rich foods	_____	(1 daily servings)
High-fat foods	_____	(2 daily servings)
Water	_____	(10 servings, 8-oz. each)

Exercise

Women who don't exercise during pregnancy become progressively less fit as the journey continues, because their bodies are becoming heavier. Exercise can counterbalance this effect and prepare your body for the physical exertion of labor and delivery while building your self-esteem and self-confidence.

Benefits of Exercise

- Increases your ability to process and utilize oxygen, enhancing transportation of oxygen and nutrients to your baby.
- Decreases risk of varicose veins, hemorrhoids, and fluid retention.
- Prevents and relieves backache and constipation.
- Makes it easier to carry added weight.
- Builds endurance so you are prepared for labor.
- Burns calories, lessens fatigue, promotes a better night's sleep.
- Imparts a feeling of confidence and increases self-esteem.

First Obtain Clearance from Your Doctor!

If you're an avid athlete, talk to your doctor about your exercise program and restructure it so it is safe for your changing body and for the baby.

If you've never exercised on a regular basis before, ask your doctor to help you choose an easy program that any novice can do:

- Walking is the easiest. You can do it anywhere—in malls, neighborhood sidewalks, and parks, even in the halls of your office building.
- Swimming.
- Riding stationary cycles.
- Calisthenics program designed especially for pregnant women.

Pulse Rate

Your pulse should not exceed 140 beats per minute for more than fifteen minutes. To figure heart rate, put your index and middle finger on the pulse point at your wrist or neck. Watch the second hand of a watch or count the pulse beats for 10 seconds. Multiply number of pulse beats times six; this number equals your heart rate.

Check your heart rate frequently during exercise as well as before and after.

Getting Started

- First, get your doctor's approval, then choose the best type of pregnancy-specific exercise program to fit yours needs.
- Equip yourself with correct and safe equipment. Wear well-cushioned shoes. Choose layered clothing for temperature adjustments.
- Stay cool while exercising. Choose times and places that are appropriate. If it's raining, snowing, or in the heat of summer, walk in a mall instead of outside.
- Eat, drink, and go to the bathroom fifteen to thirty minutes before exercising.
- Set a specific time for exercise. Build it into your schedule and set weekly goals.
- Start slowly, gradually working your way up to thirty minutes a day.
- Warm up your body before exercising. Cool down when exercise is completed.

Just Do It!
—Nike

- Exercise in moderation. Never work to a level of exhaustion.
- Remember, as your bulk increases, your balance decreases.
- Taper off your level of intensity in last trimester.
- Be prepared for the muscular aches and pains associated with any exercise program. It's a sign your hard work is paying off.

Know When to Stop!
Watch for These Warning Signs:
- Pain anywhere.
- Cramping or a stitch in your side.
- Dizziness.
- Severe breathlessness.
- Headache.
- Swelling in hands, feet, or face.
- Decrease of fetal movement.

During Exercise, Avoid—
- Pointing toes. Always flex to prevent leg cramping.
- Pulling of abdominal muscles (sit-ups, leg lifts, front stretches).
- Overextending joints of the knee, ankle, or elbow.
- Lying flat on back.
- Quick changes in direction, jumping, vigorous and straining movements
- Weight-bearing or lifting exercises.
- Hot or humid weather.

Record in Your Journal Each Time You Exercise
- When you have your doctor's okay, set a weekly goal for yourself.
- Promise: *I will exercise 4 times a week for at least 30 minutes a day.*

When You Can't Exercise
Even if your doctor has restricted your physical exercise, you can exercise your mind and spirit instead. Use the scheduled exercise period as a *quiet time* of reflection and relaxation. Choose a subject-specific Bible study in an area related to parenting or character development. Learning to meditate will teach your mind to focus on a task, increase body awareness, and help meet the challenges of childbirth and motherhood.

Don't Forget to Do Your Kegels Every Day!
Kegel exercises are a simple way to strengthen the vaginal and perineal area in preparation for delivery. To do a Kegel, tense the muscles around vagina and anus for as long as you can hold them, then slowly release the muscles and relax. A good drill is to work the muscles, tensing up for a count of eight, then slowly releasing, counting down from eight to one. Kegels can be done while standing, sitting, or urinating. Try to complete twenty-five Kegels through your day. If you do a few of these toning exercises at every red traffic light, you will be preparing your body for the labor of giving birth.

Insurance Information and Billing Policy

My medical insurance company is _____

My medical insurance phone number is _____

My policy number is _____

    Now is the time to take a hard look at your medical insurance. To make sure medical expenses will not bring bad surprises, find answers to the following questions:

What is my deductible? $ _____

What percent of my covered medical expenses is reimbursed? $ _____

What percent do I pay? $ _____

What is my out-of-pocket expense cap? $ _____

WHAT PERCENT IS COVERED OF—

Prenatal care visits? _____

Prenatal tests? _____

Vitamins and prescriptions? _____

Genetic counseling? _____

Standard delivery? _____

Cesarean delivery? _____

Well-baby care in hospital? _____

Neonatal complications? _____

Nursery care in hospital? _____

Services of a licensed midwife? _____

Delivery at a birthing center or non-hospital environment? _____

Is the baby covered at birth? _____

How many well-baby visits are covered? _____

Baby's immunizations? _____

How many hospital days allowed for a vaginal delivery? _____

How many hospital days allowed for a cesarean delivery? _____

Answers to other specific questions about my medical coverage:

_____

_____

_____

_____

    Find out the specifics of what you are responsible to pay. Make an appointment with your doctor's office manager and find out what, when, and how you will be billed.

Answers to specific questions about my doctor's billing policy:

_____

_____

_____

_____

Record of Medical Expenses

Use this reference chart to keep track of all your prenatal medical expenses and reimbursements.

Date	Doctor or pharmacy	How Paid	Amount	Amount Toward deductible	Amount Insurance paid	Amount we paid	Date Reimbursed	Total we paid

Medical insurance company is _____

Medical insurance phone number is _____

Policy number is _____

Notes

The Budget

The birth of a child is a life-altering event that affects the mind, body, soul, and wallet. You're preparing yourself for all the changes that your body, mind, and life will undergo on your journey. Don't forget to prepare your finances and plan for future expenditures. *Begin saving!*

Medical Expenses

No matter how good your health insurance, the birth of a child will cost you something extra. Work through the "Insurance Information and Billing Policy" (page 120) and educate yourself on what you are expected to pay. Keep filling in your "Record of Medical Expenses" (page 121).

For information on local medical financial aid programs and prenatal support, look in your area phone book.

Maternity Clothes

The sky's the limit on how much you can spend or borrow from friends. I suggest that instead of buying a whole wardrobe in the fourth month, start with the basics. Add something new every month. With this method, you can give yourself a monthly budget for buying. If you don't spend the stash on maternity clothes, save it for something else like a mother's pamper day at the salon or a special gift for the baby.

Outfitting the Nursery

With your calculator and a notepad in hand, take a stroll through your local baby store or the baby section of a department store. You'll quickly see that all the little necessities add up quickly. Decide how much you are able to spend. Start putting money aside now. You may want to borrow some things from friends or relatives. Research equipment to be sure it is safe.

Last-Fling Vacation

You don't have to go to Paris for vacation, but if possible try to plan for a getaway in the fifth or sixth month. Get your doctor's permission. After working on "The Budget Chart" (pages 123-124), decide how much you can afford and plan your destination accordingly.

Baby's Layette

There are definite necessities—diapers, formula, clothes, blankets—you must have for the baby. Borrow where appropriate. Let a friend plan a shower. Make a list, and set a budget to buy the remaining items on the list.

Childcare and Baby's Education

You need to start thinking about who will care for baby if you go back to work. Adjust your post-baby budget to accommodate childcare costs. You also need to establish a savings fund for your baby's education. Commit yourself to contributing to that fund monthly.

Income Replacement During Maternity Leave

Find out what your maternity-leave benefits are. Decide how much time you want to take off. Thanks to the Family Leave Act, you are entitled by law to take 12 weeks of leave. Most companies pay for 6 to 8 weeks. If you want to stay home longer, discuss this with your boss. Then start saving to replace the lost income.

The Budget Chart

It's time to pull your calculator out, put pencil to paper, and start financial planning for your baby. This exercise will walk you through a simple monthly budget and help you evaluate if you need to start putting some money aside for the things you deem important and how much you should save.

ITEM	OLD BUDGET	NEW BUDGET
Father's salary	$_____	$_____
Mother's salary	_____	_____
Interest income	_____	_____
Dividends	_____	_____
Capital Gains	_____	_____
Other income	_____	_____
TOTAL MONTHLY INCOME	$_____	_____
Rent or mortgage payments	$_____	$_____
Car payments, transportation costs	_____	_____
Insurance (auto, home, health, life)	_____	_____
Loan payments	_____	_____
Tithes	_____	_____
Utilities for the home	_____	_____
Phone costs	_____	_____
TV cable and Internet connection	_____	_____
Childcare during working hours	_____	_____
TOTAL FIXED EXPENSES	$_____	$_____
Auto gas and maintenance	$_____	$_____
Allowances and walking-around money	_____	_____
Bank or credit union charges	_____	_____
Charitable contributions (beyond tithes)	_____	_____
Childcare after working hours	_____	_____
Clothing	_____	_____
Credit cards	_____	_____
Loan # 1 payments	_____	_____
Loan # 2 payments	_____	_____
Entertainment, dining out, travel	_____	_____
Fitness and beauty	_____	_____
Gifts	_____	_____
Groceries	_____	_____
Laundry, dry cleaning	_____	_____
Medical costs paid by family	_____	_____
Repairs, servicing, disasters	_____	_____
Savings	_____	_____
Miscellaneous	_____	_____
TOTAL FLEXIBLE EXPENSES	$_____	$_____

Medical expenses extra for pregnancy	$_____	_____
Maternity clothes	_____	_____
Outfitting the nursery	_____	_____
Vacation for parents-to-be	_____	_____
Baby's layette	_____	_____
Income replacement for maternity leave	_____	_____
Childcare, baby's education	_____	_____
Other added expenses	_____	_____
TOTAL BABY EXPENSES	$_____	$_____

SUMMARY

Total Monthly Income	$_____	$_____
Minus Total Fixed Expenses	_____	_____
Minus Total Flexible Expenses	_____	_____
Minus Total Baby Expenses	_____	_____
Money Remaining	_____	_____
OR Shortfall	_____	_____

REDUCTIONS OR RESOURCES TO MANAGE ANY SHORTFALL

_____

_____

_____

_____

_____

_____

_____

_____

_____

_____

_____

_____

_____

_____

_____

_____

_____

Those who gather little by little will increase wealth,
and those who spend a little less here and a little less there, will also increase it.
Proverbs 13:11, expanded

The Author

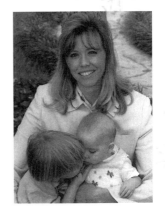

*J*ESSICA Lee Kelly is the mother of two boys, Colton and Clayton. She is married to Michael, a commercial airline pilot, and they live near Fort Worth. Kelly's pre-mom life includes a marketing degree from Texas A & M University, a buying career in retail for two nationwide department stores, and a passion for quiet Saturdays with mornings of sleeping in and afternoons of lounging by the pool. Now Saturdays are filled with the toughest job she'll ever love—motherhood.

Nevertheless, Kelly still finds time to attend Bible Study Fellowship International, teach Bible study at Celebration Baptist Church, where she and Michael are members, and write articles for the church newsletter.

Word pictures have marked great and small landmarks in Kelly's life. From childhood, she has kept a journal, which God has used to reveal his presence and to build her faith that the Lord is indeed working every day in her life.

Kelly was raised by parents who nurtured her relationship with God. She accepted Christ as Savior and Lord, then helplessly watched her mother fight a three-year losing battle with cancer. For several teenage years, she struggled before learning there was no place God would let her go alone. God's Spirit was always there, ready to forgive and bless once she turned back to the Lord. In her twenties, Kelly celebrated her homecoming to faith by using God's gift for writing. Stories poured out. Her letters, essays, and fiction led to winning a writing contest.

Then in her thirties, she came full circle from grief into the miraculous season of motherhood. Her time for writing was limited. In her journal she composed short essays on life walked by faith. Storytelling turned into monthly letters treasured by friends and family. One of her family Christmas letters was published in Mary L. Schramski's book *Love Letters* (Rainbow Books).

One day in 1995, Kelly prayed, "Lord, what do you want me to write today?" God's answer was *The Miracle Journey*. She believes God has a purpose for this book that is greater than her own thoughts. Christian women are searching for growth, guidance, and companionship on this journey, just as she was in spiritual development during pregnancy.

Jessica Lee Kelly's prayer each morning is that she will seize the day and live it joyously, giving others a testimony of the grace and love of Christ.

More Journal Notes